Program Planning
Health Education
Health Promotion

Program Planning for Health Education and Health Promotion

Mark B. Dignan, Ph.D., M.P.H.
Associate Professor
Department of Family and Community
Medicine
Bowman Gray School of Medicine
Wake Forest University
Winston-Salem, North Carolina

Patricia A. Carr, M.P.H.
Lecturer, Department of Public
Health Education
University of North Carolina at Greensboro
Greensboro, North Carolina

Lea & Febiger *Philadelphia*

1987

Lea & Febiger
600 Washington Square
Philadelphia, PA 19106
U.S.A.

Library of Congress Cataloging-in-Publication Data

Dignan, Mark B.
  Program planning for health education and health
promotion.

  Rev. ed. of: Introduction to program planning. 1981.
  Includes bibliographies and index.
  1. Health education—Planning.   2. Health promotion—
Planning.   3. Community health services—Planning.
I. Carr, Patricia A.   II. Dignan, Mark B.   Introduction
to program planning.   III. Title.   [DNLM: 1. Health
Education.   2. Health Planning.   3. Health Promotion.
WA 590 D575i]
RA440.5.D55   1987   613'.07   87-3937
ISBN 0-8121-1091-9

PRINTED IN THE UNITED STATES OF AMERICA

Print Number: 3   2   1

FOR

Allison, Laurel Anna, Randy, and Stephen

Foreword

Community health education program planning, the focus of this book, can be said to have two historical roots. The first might be termed the early community studies literature, and the second, the planned change literature.

For many years, community health education practice was guided and informed by these two categories of scientific and professional literature. It is only relatively recently that a new genre of texts directed at organizing and rationalizing health education program planning and evaluation has emerged. This genre includes books that attempt to develop program planning and evaluation models, and books of health education case studies.

The earlier literature was characterized by a certain richness and depth of understanding of communities. The current health education program planning and evaluation texts have drawn upon these earlier works as well as on systems theory, social research methods, health planning, and epidemiology for their conceptual and theoretic frameworks. Collectively and individually, these books are making an important contribution to the further development and advancement of the practice of community health education.

This book is a welcome addition to this growing and important category of texts. The authors present the basic elements of community health education program planning and evaluation in six comprehensive chapters. An overall model of the program planning process is presented and explained in Chapter 1. This model is then used as the conceptual framework for the book. Each chapter elaborates on one component of the model and provides the information necessary to complete a stage of the planning process.

The text has many strengths, and I would like to point out those that seem particularly noteworthy. Most program planning texts specify the steps to be taken in the planning process, but few ever specify who is to accomplish them. In Chapter 1, Dignan and Carr plainly say that the planning process is a collaborative endeavor between the professional and the client community. Communities are not treated as passive entitites for which plans are developed and on which subsequent programs are inflicted. Rather, they are treated as active partners in the program planning, implementation, and evaluation processes. This is an important concept; first, because it is the only practical way to ensure the development of effective programs and their acceptance by client communities; second, because it distinguishes health education program planning from other types of health planning.

Chapter 2, "Community Analysis," defines the concept of community and then presents a comprehensive format for conducting a community analysis. This analysis includes geographic, social, political, economic, epidemiologic, and health service components. In a few informative pages, the authors have included all of the key elements of a comprehensive community analysis. Any health education student or practitioner can easily refer to this chapter to see what should be included in a comprehensive community analysis. In my opinion, the book is worth its cost for this chapter alone.

Chapter 3 concerns the focus of the program. This chapter includes important concepts such as determining community-felt needs, defining target behaviors, and establishing program goals and objectives. The chapter is based on sound, up-to-date health education theory and principles, which should be of use to any health professional planning a program.

Chapters 4 and 5 cover development and implementation of a program plan.

The final chapter, 6, which concerns evaluation, is also comprehensive. A health professional planning a program could review this chapter and know what elements should be included in his or her evaluation plan. The chapter presents five levels of evaluation: activity, minimum standards, efficiency, effectiveness, outcome, and appropriateness. The chapter also discusses the basic evaluation designs that are most commonly used in health education, i.e., nonequivalent control group; pretest, posttest; and post-test only. Threats to validity, and other strengths and weaknesses of each of these designs are discussed.

I was particularly impressed with the inclusion of qualitative evaluation methods in this chapter. Dignan and Carr recognize that in health education and promotion not all program effects can be precisely measured. In such cases, the use of qualitative methods is warranted. Through participant observations and interviews, evaluators can carefully document program implementation. Such documentation frequently can be useful in helping to explain quantitative evaluation results. This book makes an important contribution to health education and promotion through suggesting a combined quantitative and qualitative approach to program evaluation.

Allan Steckler, Dr.P.H.
Associate Professor
Department of Health Education
School of Public Health
University of North Carolina,
Chapel Hill

Preface

Since the publication in 1981 of INTRODUCTION TO PROGRAM PLAN-NING: A BASIC TEXT FOR COMMUNITY HEALTH EDUCATION, we have witnessed tremendous growth in health education in this country and around the world. This growth has created a much more complex field. When we were preparing the manuscript for that first book, our conception of planning, implementation, and evaluation of health education programs focused on the activities of health education practitioners, the identification of health problems in specific target populations, and the development of plans for education programs. This approach was pragmatic and useful at that time, but perhaps is overly simplistic today. In the years since, health education has expanded in breadth and complexity. Quite naturally, the process of program planning has expanded concomitantly.

In preparing this manuscript, we have based our work on an expanded view of health education that can be summarized in three "guiding principles."

First, health education now includes the concept of health promotion. Health promotion is much broader in concept than health education and involves advocacy for good health in a wide variety of ways, including education. The addition of health promotion concerns alters the traditional approach to program planning to a great extent. We have made, therefore, several important changes in our earlier work. On the most general level, we have broadened our perspective to include the health promotion point of view. We have added examples, using health promotion to illustrate important principles, and have reoriented much of the material in our earlier work to accomodate the concept of health promotion. We have applied this principle throughout the text, but it is most visible in the first three chapters in which assessment for planning is discussed.

Second, in considering the planning process, it is clear that health educators are only one group among numerous health professionals who are involved with the planning, implementation, and evaluation of health education and health promotion programs. We have reconstructed much of the text to include the wide variety of health professionals who are now involved in program planning for health education and health promotion. The addition of these "new" health professionals—nurses, nutritionists, environmental health specialists, classroom teachers, physicians, and others—into the planning process brings additional useful points of view into the process. The influence of these points of view is felt most keenly in the assessment that is carried out prior to planning.

Third, well conceived evaluation of health education / promotion programs continues to grow in importance. As the emphasis on preventing disease continues to gain momentum, critical assessment of the effectiveness of programs that espouse prevention as a goal also gains importance. To accomodate the increasing emphasis on evaluation, as well as the complexity of the subject itself, the chapter on evaluation has been completely restructured. The chapter begins with a review of the basic theory of evaluation, including the qualitative approach. Following this introduction, the theory is applied to evaluation of health education and promotion programs. In general, we have made evaluation perhaps the most comprehensive chapter in the text.

One of the strengths of our earlier work was its clear language. We have struggled to retain that feature in this manuscript, while broadening our perspective and discussing many topics in greater depth. We firmly believe that program planning is an applied activity that is done well when people communicate with one another effectively. With communication in mind, we have attempted to put forth our ideas clearly and simply, at the expense of occasionally short-cutting detailed explanations of processes and activities. In order to fill the need for such explanations, we have selected references for the end of each chapter that supply additional detail, in addition to fulfilling the traditional function of references of supporting assertions of fact.

Mark B. Dignan

Patricia A. Carr

Acknowledgments

We were very fortunate to have had the generous services of the individuals listed below in providing the professional review that was needed for preparation of this manuscript. We thank them for their help.

Mohammed Forouzesh
California State University, Long Beach
Long Beach, California

David Foulk
University of Florida
Gainesville, Florida

Mildred Kaufman
School of Public Health
University of North Carolina
Chapel Hill, North Carolina

Allan Steckler
School of Public Health
University of North Carolina
Chapel Hill, North Carolina

The staff at Lea & Febiger have been continually supportive and helpful to us. We appreciated the talent and patience of Tanya Lazar, who assisted us in making numerous editorial decisions, and of George Mundorff, our editor, who continually supported and encouraged us.

Finally, we would like to acknowledge the following individuals who contributed in many different ways to the earlier version of this text, INTRODUCTION TO PROGRAM PLANNING: A BASIC TEXT FOR COMMUNITY HEALTH EDUCATION: Guy Steuart, JoAnne Earp, Stuart Marks, Robert Kane, F. David Fisher, Charles Hughes, Marshall Kreuter, Thomas Mackey, Richard Dwore, Irshad Ahmad, Alton Wilson, Karin Rolett, Bob Robinson, Diane Bergeron, Mary Wooten, Janice Beaver, Marla Rutter, Jeff Gilliam, Donna Winchell, Susan McBane, Karen King, Scott Lawrence, Rosemary Nelson, Genie Sloan, Pheon Beal, Thomasin Bradford, Lynn Knapp, Jean Eastwood, Alan Michael, and Margaret Thompson.

Mark B. Dignan
Patricia A. Carr

Contents

Chapter 1   Program Planning; Putting the Parts Together   3
             Basic Definitions and Assumptions   4
             Theoretical Foundations   6
             Targets of Program Planning   10
             Process of Program Planning   12
Chapter 2   Community Analysis   17
             Understanding Communities   18
             Involvement of Health Professionals   19
             Format for Community Analysis   19
             Collecting Data from the Community   46
Chapter 3   Focusing Program Development   53
             Extending Community Analysis   53
             Establishing Program Goals   56
             Defining Target Group Behaviors   58
             Models for Behavioral Assessment   61
             Methods for Collecting Data on Health Behaviors
                 and Outcomes   67
             Assessing Educational Readiness   70
             Determining Program Focus   74
Chapter 4   Developing a Program Plan   85
             Components of Program Plans   85
             The Planning Process   85
             Creating the Planning Document   99
             Examples of Program Plans 103
Chapter 5   Program Implementation 113
             Phases of Implementation 114
             Using Planned Procedures to Produce Changes in the
                 Target Population 122
Chapter 6   Program Evaluation 127
             Scope of Evaluation 128
             Focus of Program Evaluation 131
             Sources of Evaluation 132
             Criteria for Evaluation 133
             Measurement and Evaluation 135
             Evaluation Design 139
             Quantitative Evaluation 143
             Qualitative Evaluation 147
             Combined Quantitative and Qualitative Methods 148
             Planning for Evaluation 149
             Accountability and Program Evaluation 151
Index   157

Program Planning for Health Education and Health Promotion

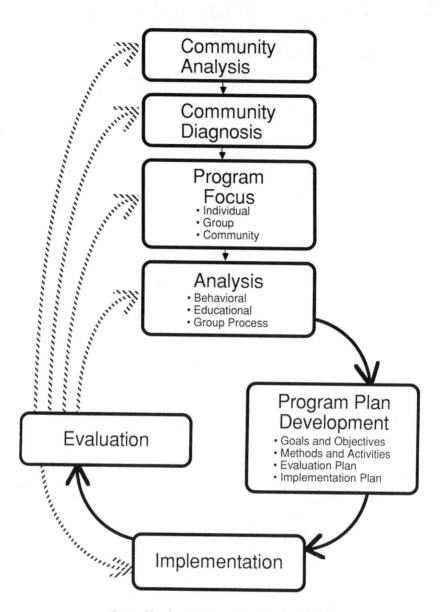

The Health Education/Promotion Planning Model.

1

Program Planning; Putting the Parts Together

Effective planning requires communication, cooperation, and coordination between those persons who provide and those persons who receive services, as well as among those individuals who plan for service delivery. A useful way of illustrating this concept is to review the childhood tale about the blind men and the elephant.[1]

Six blind men who lived in India had often heard about elephants, but obviously had never seen one, so they went to the palace of the Rajah to "see" an elephant. They explored the elephant individually, touching various parts of the animal with their hands. On the basis of their experiences, each man came up with a unique idea of what an elephant must be like. The first man, feeling the side of the elephant, thought it must be like a wall; the second man, finding the trunk, thought an elephant was like a snake; and the third man, feeling the tusk, thought the animal was like a spear. The fourth man, discovering the elephant's leg, thought it resembled a tree; the fifth man, feeling the ear, believed the animal was flat and shaped like a fan; and the sixth man, at the tail, thought the elephant was like a rope. After the blind men had finished their explorations, each tried to convince the others that he alone had the correct perception of what the elephant was like. It soon became clear that each man's description was so different that there was little point in trying to convince the others. The blind men were confused. An observer, watching and listening to the debate, finally told the six blind men that the elephant is a huge animal, and that each description was accurate for only a small part. The observer advised the men to put their descriptions together. The blind men proceeded to discuss the parts of the elephant, and each man finally came to an understanding of what an elephant is like.

The connection between the story and program planning lies in the relationship between seemingly unrelated parts of a whole and how they can be put together to form a complete picture. The blind men had a clear notion of their goal—to find out about elephants. Being blind, however, they had to rely on information from other sources (one another) to reach that goal. Most importantly, however, by using that newly acquired information, they showed a willingness to revise their thinking about the elephant. Individuals involved in planning health education and promotion programs are usually in a position much like that of the blind men. The impetus for planning is a need to "see" something that is beyond our vision, for example, new health services or the means to promote healthy lifestyles. Planning designed to meet this need necessitates collecting information about the need as well as about how it might be met. Analysis of the information collected enables us to "see" only if our original ideas may be changed based on new information.

As an illustration, suppose a notion is put forth that community residents need more exercise. This idea may seem straightforward initially, but the clarity disappears when the details are considered. To plan effectively, clear and specific descriptions of all goals are needed. Does the phrase "need more exercise" mean people will exercise more for some specific reason or just for the overall benefits that are associated with exercise? Is there a particular form of exercise in mind? Is the target a particular group of community citizens? Is the exercise aerobic in nature? The list of questions goes on and on. The point is that, like the blind men, we often begin to conceptualize health education and promotion without clear goals; our vision develops and improves as we progress through the planning process. Just as sorting out the varied descriptions of the parts brought the blind men to a clearer understanding of the elephant, careful planning helps to clarify and to integrate the parts needed to produce a focused, coherent program of health education and promotion.

BASIC DEFINITIONS AND ASSUMPTIONS

Planning is an unconscious act that occurs every day of our lives. Accordingly, whether the plan involves what to eat for lunch or how to increase public knowledge of risk factors for heart disease, certain features are common to most of our thoughts and actions. Effective planning requires anticipation of what will be needed along the way to reaching a goal. This statement implies that the goal is defined, as are the necessary steps, or parts, involved in reaching the goal. Perhaps most importantly, it requires an understanding of the parts (steps) themselves and how they interrelate.

Health education and health promotion are usually presented as *programs*. Interpreting the meaning of the term program has become a challenge in itself, and in some sense, the term is now overused and does not convey much meaning at all. To "program" in the sense of computer programming, however, is a useful analogy for our discussion, because a computer program is literally a set of statements intended to define the functions of the machine so that it will produce a specific outcome. When the term program is used in health education and promotion, the meaning is similar: program is a package of services, information, or both that is intended to produce a particular result. Programs usually require specific and clear goals and objectives, combined with reasonable and appropriate methods for satisfying the objectives and thereby reaching the goals. Evaluation should figure prominently in such programs, along with methods for implementation. One of the central purposes of this book is to describe how programs are planned, and how the results of planning can be expressed through program plans. *Program plans* are sets of statements (that usually become documents) that describe a package of services intended to accomplish a particular purpose. The details regarding the development of program plans are recounted in Chapter 4.

Health education is education intended to have a positive impact on health. In our view, health includes physical, emotional, social, and value-oriented aspects, so health education can properly be directed toward positive changes in one or any combination of these areas of concern. In addition, in addressing these aspects of health, health education may be intentionally directed toward knowledge levels, attitudes, or specific behaviors.

Health promotion is a broad concept and includes providing health education and information intended to promote health. Promoting health involves advocating increased awareness of personal and community health, changing attitudes so that changes in behavior are possible, and searching for alternatives to improve health.[2]

Two basic assumptions bear on all of the aforementioned definitions. First, we believe that people not only have the right, but also the responsibility to participate in planning health education and promotion programs that are intended to influence them. Accordingly, the population for whom planning is done is urged to become involved on as many levels as possible. Our bias makes sense; people are more eager to adopt changes when they play a role in determining what the changes will be and how they will be effected. Second, we acknowledge that health education and health promotion are provided by many different types of health providers. Health educators are usually involved primarily with the planning, implementation, and evaluation of health services; however, nurses, nutritionists, physical therapists, occupational therapists, social workers, volunteers in health-related service organizations and institutions, and many other individuals may also be involved in delivering services. No single profession has a corner on the delivery of health education or health promotion. Physicians and dentists play a central role in the delivery of health education and promotion; the care they provide often includes education and information, and they are also a primary source of referral to programs of various types.

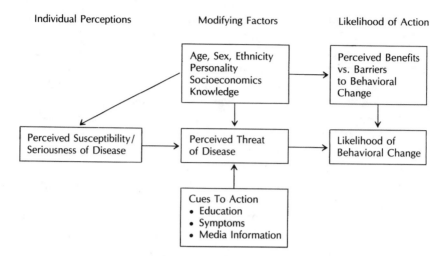

Fig. 1–1. Components of the Health Belief Model. (Adapted from Rosenstock, I. M.: Historical origins of the Health Belief Model. *In* The Health Belief Model and Personal Health Behavior. Edited by M. H. Becker. Thorofare, N.J., Charles B. Slack, 1974.)

THEORETICAL FOUNDATIONS

Planning requires understanding of the parts of programs and how they are intended to interact to produce an outcome. The driving force producing this understanding is theory. Theoretical guidance for health education and promotion has for the most part been borrowed from other disciplines, including social and behavioral psychology, communication theory, and most recently, social marketing. Detailed description of these disciplines is beyond the scope of this discussion. The focus instead is on the application of theory with the use of models formulated to help understand and predict health behaviors and mechanisms for producing change. Models are presented that address three tasks that are basic to program planning for health education and promotion. First, the Health Belief Model provides a model for analyzing the forces that impact health behavior. Second, the Communication/Persuasion Matrix and the Communication/Behavior-Change Framework add important elements of communication theory to the development of education directed to produce behavioral change. Third, the Social Marketing Framework provides guidance for program design and development of strategies to introduce programs effectively to the target population.

Health Belief Model

This model was formulated in the 1950s, and was based on experience with public participation in a screening program for tuberculosis.[3] Analysis of the various forces and factors that influenced participation resulted in the development of the model (Fig. 1–1).[4, 5]

The Health Belief Model is based on three essential factors: (1) the readiness of the individual to consider behavioral changes to avoid disease or to minimize health risks; (2) the existence and power of forces in the individual's environment that urge change and make it possible; and (3) the behaviors themselves. Each of these factors is influenced by a complex set of forces that relate to the personality and environment of the individual, as well as past experiences with health services and providers.

The readiness of the individual is influenced by forces that include perception of vulnerability to disease, potency of the threat, motivation for reducing vulnerability, and extent of the belief that behavioral change will be beneficial. Forces that influence behavioral change are themselves influenced by the personal characteristics of the individual, the appraisal by the individual of the extent of the changes proposed, the effects of interactions with the health professionals recommending change, and previous experiences with similar attempts at behavioral change.

The Health Belief Model may be involved in program planning in two ways: by providing first an outline of the essential factors involved in behavioral change, and second, a guide to careful exploration of the personality and environment of the target (individual, group, or community). Both of these aspects help the health professional to understand better how to plan programs that deal effectively with impediments to change.

Communication / Persuasion Matrix

Although the focus of the Health Belief Model is on the personal, social, and psychologic factors related to behavioral change, the specific impact of communication on the process of change is not considered. The focus of the Communication / Persuasion Matrix is on the process of change; the matrix provides a format for evaluating the impact of various types of communication on that process (Fig. 1–2).[6] The 12 items listed on the left margin of Figure 1–2 set forth a sequence of events that occur during the process of behavioral change. The characteristics of communication are listed on the horizontal axis. "Source" refers to the characteristics of the individual or the organization that is perceived to be delivering the communication. The choice of a source depends on the result desired. A source with high credibility, such as a physician, is best suited for an educational goal, such as encouraging the practice of breast self-examination. For another goal, however, such as promoting exercise for fitness, an obviously physically fit source demonstrating the desired behavior would be a good choice. "Message" denotes the content of the communication. Education may be packaged in messages that are short, long, simple, or complicated, the type depending on the goals involved. To attract community residents to a screening program, the message might be short and simple. For those persons suspected of having the disease, information about follow-up care might be more detailed.

Elements of the Process of Behavioral Change	Communication Characteristics				
	Source	Message	Channel	Receiver	Destination
1. Exposure to education					
2. Attention to education					
3. Interest in new information					
4. Comprehension of education					
5. Acquisition of new skills					
6. Attitude change					
7. Memory of skills					
8. Recall of skills					
9. Decision to change					
10. Action (behavior change)					
11. Reinforcement					
12. Re-affirmation of change					

Fig. 1-2.   The Communication / Persuasion Matrix. (Adapted from McGuire, W. J.: Theoretical foundations of campaigns. *In* Public Communication Campaigns. Edited by R. E. Rice and W. J. Paisley. Beverly Hills, Sage, 1981.)

FUNCTIONS OF SENDER OF COMMUNICATION	OBJECTIVES FOR BEHAVIORAL CHANGE IN RECEIVER
1. Gain attention / set agenda	1. Become aware
2. Provide information	2. Increase knowledge
3. Clarify incentives	3. Increase motivation
4. Model behaviors	4. Learn skills
5. Provide training	5. Use skills to change
6. Cues to action	6. Incorporate change into lifestyle
7. Provide support	7. Maintain changed behaviors

Fig. 1–3.   Elements of the Communication / Behavior-Change Framework.

"Channel" is the medium through which the message is communicated. Typical channels are verbal, audiovisual, and printed. Each type of communication has its own strengths and weaknesses.

"Receiver" refers to important characteristics of the person who receives the communication. Age, ethnicity, and socioeconomic status are potentially important factors, but the ability to use the information in the context of present and past experiences with health problems may dramatically affect the way that information is received. Any characteristic that is likely to influence how the information is received should be considered in planning.

"Destination" refers to the anticipated impact of the communication on the receiver in light of the change that is anticipated. The change may be short or long term, simple or complex.

The Communication / Persuasion Matrix can be used to assist in program planning by breaking the process of change into components and pointing out ways of matching the mode and style of communication to the desired behavioral change.

Communication / Behavior-Change (CBC) Framework

The CBC Framework is a combination of the concepts of the Health Belief Model and an adapted version of the Communication / Persuasion Matrix that yields a means for developing community-based health education and promotion programs (Fig. 1–3).[7] This framework was developed for use in planning educational programs as part of community-based research on prevention of cardiovascular disease (The Stanford Three Community Study).[8] Functions for the provider of the education are paired with objectives for change in the targets. This approach may be useful to the program planner in helping to develop realistic objectives for behavior change in the target population and in developing specific educational strategies to reach the objectives. Specifically, the functions that need planning are as follows:

Agenda setting. Gain the attention of community residents and attract attention to the issues to be addressed by the program.

Information. Present information in terms that can be understood by community residents and that in turn predisposes them to behavioral change.

Incentives. Present information that clearly identifies the benefits that may be realized through changing behaviors.

Models. Demonstrate necessary skills.

Training. Provide education that teaches use of new skills.

Cues to action. Provide reminders to the public to keep the recommended change in focus.

Support. Promote maintenance of behavioral change through creation of a sense of community among residents.

Social Marketing Framework

Social marketing is the use of the principles and techniques of marketing to increase the effectiveness of programs designed to produce social change.[9] Specifically, social marketing is the design, implementation, and control of programs seeking to increase the acceptability of a social idea or cause in a target group(s)."[7] Programs to promote healthy lifestyles or to teach specific changes in health behavior fit under the rubric of social programs.

The marketing process can be summarized by the "four Ps of marketing management: the right PRODUCT backed by the right PROMOTION and put in the right PLACE at the right PRICE."[7] For health education and promotion, the product is the program. To be marketed successfully, the program must be developed with the needs and interests of the target population clearly in mind. The promotion component is the means for making the program visible and attractive. Place relates to the understanding by the target population of the means and logistics involved in obtaining program services. The fourth component, price, relates to the cost of participation in the program. Cost may be expressed in many ways, including money, time, or energy. Programs that are received well by the target populations are promoted by using clear statements about the relationship between costs and benefits for the participants.[8] The Health Belief Model, the Communication / Persuasion Matrix, the Communication / Behavior-Change Framework, and the Social Marketing Framework provide elements of a foundation for planning health education and promotion programs. It is important to remember, however, that because of the variety of program needs, the utility of the models is in the conceptual frameworks provided for planning, and not in guidance for meeting specific needs. In each situation, careful analysis of needs, interests, and concerns is required to identify the targets of education; planning can then begin.

TARGETS OF PROGRAM PLANNING

A program plan specifies behavior(s) that must be maintained or changed to bring about desired outcomes. The behaviors originate in the individual but may be more effectively changed or reinforced by programs that focus on a group or a larger system, such as a health care delivery system.

Individuals. Health education focused on specific needs of the individual often takes the form of patient education. Patient education programs often involve extensive individual interviewing and counseling for the benefit of a patient with a specific concern. Weight control programs for preventing the progression of diabetes mellitus and hypertension, for example, commonly require individual attention to the details of the lifestyle of an individual so that weight control, compliance with therapy, and other ends can be achieved. The health professional in such a setting plans an individual health education strategy to help a patient attain a specific goal.

Groups. Health professionals also plan programs that concentrate on groups of clients as the focus of change. Where individuals may benefit from a group setting, various types of group health education programs may be designed. When planning health education that focuses on the individual, the health provider can tailor program plans to accommodate most personal preferences; but when planning for groups, the efforts directed toward tailoring plans for the individual must be reconciled with the needs of the group as a whole. Health education programs that focus on groups have several benefits. Collective group behavior utilized to promote change in the individual members of the group is a by-product of such forces as peer pressure, collective decision-making, and group support. Mastectomy self-help groups, "Weight Watchers," and "Alcoholics Anonymous" are all examples of groups that provide additional support to the individual through the influence of group participation. Programs planned for groups may also cost less and require less individualized attention, less time, and fewer staff members to implement. Care must be taken, however, that these savings do not supercede the needs and desires of the target population in dictating the type of program to be planned.

Communities. Health providers may also plan health education programs that focus on change for a total health care delivery system or a geographic area. In this instance, health education functions as one component of a total program. Family planning programs, chronic disease screening programs, various school health programs, and maternal and child health programs usually include planned health education as a component of their services. In planning these programs, the health educators interact with the other health professionals involved with the program to plan a coordinated, comprehensive health care service.

The goals of a particular health education program often determine whether the individual, a group, or an entire community should be the focus of the program. The provider of the service must understand the desired health goals and related behaviors of the population, even if it is a population of one, to plan a program that facilitates and supports the process of change.

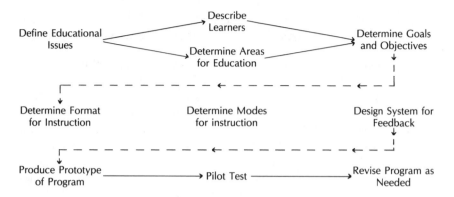

Fig. 1-4. A general model for instructional development.

PROCESS OF PROGRAM PLANNING

Planning for health education and promotion programs is based on a general, rational model for the development of education. The model sets forth the basic components needed to develop structured programs of instruction (Fig. 1–4). The specific nature of health education, however, makes adoption of this model less appropriate. To guide planning, a model is needed that includes not only the components of instructional development, but also guidance for the development of programs attuned to the special needs and interests related to health.

Given the theories related to health beliefs, communication, and social marketing principles, as well as the need for sensitivity to health-related needs and interests, we developed a model for planning health education and promotion programs; the essential components of the planning process are shown in the figure at the beginning of this chapter. We purposely refer to program planning as a process, because, when properly executed, it involves a continuous cycle of assessment, development of educational and promotional strategies, implementation, and evaluation.[10–12]

The process of program planning for community health education comprises a series of interconnected steps: (1) community analysis, (2) community diagnosis, (3) establishment of program focus, (4) target (group) analysis, (5) program plan development, (6) implementation, and (7) evaluation.

Community Analysis. Community analysis involves the collection of detailed information concerning the community under study. After a general overview is obtained, specific aspects of the community are analyzed, including the general health status, the health care system, and the social assistance system. Information required for the analysis is derived from a variety of sources. Some of the information can be found in official documents from national, state, or local agencies. Collection of information reflecting internal functions of the community usually requires use of special techniques to determine how and why communities function as they do.

Community Diagnosis. Community diagnosis, the final step in community analysis, involves the synthesis of collected data and the identification of gaps between health problems and services. The gaps are indications of need within the community and of any subpopulations that may be particularly affected by health problems. This group or groups become the target population(s) for health education programming. When health gaps and target populations have been identified by community analysis, it is essential that any indicated need be perceived and verified by the target population.

Establishment of Program Focus. Once the needs are verified, all subsequent activities in the program planning process for health education focus on designing a program that is oriented to a specific target population with identified needs. Community analysis may identify a need that cannot be alleviated through health education intervention. For example, the community need may be addressed most appropriately through a medical services program. On the other hand, a need may be identified for which health education, either alone or in conjunction with other intervention strategies, is the appropriate and desired approach to resolution.

Target (Group) Analysis. If health education intervention is indicated, it is necessary to define behaviors related to the problem. The essence of health education is planned behavior change—planned changes in behaviors that are related to maintenance and improvement of health. To effect this change, the program plan must be based on the findings derived from a thorough assessment of current behaviors of the target population. In health education, behavior assessment involves procedures derived from two main sources, social psychology and behavioral psychology.

The social psychology perspective focuses on factors in the environment, including other people, that predispose the occurrence of behavior, enable a behavior to be performed or maintained, and/or provide reinforcement. Interactions of individuals or groups with the society in which they live and work gives rise to these factors; hence the reference to a social-psychologic perspective.

The behavioral psychology perspective focuses more directly on behaviors themselves, as well as the specific mechanisms that maintain or suppress behaviors. These behaviors are usually linked, and often an entire sequence of behaviors is included as the focus for assessment. Assessment from the behavioral psychology perspective includes consideration of the role of stimuli that precede behavior, factors related to the physiologic state of the organism that relate to the behavior, the nature of the behavior itself, and the long and short-term consequences of the behavior.

Use of these two perspectives in assessing behavior provides the health professional planning a program with an image of the behaviors to be changed, including an individual as well as a societal dimension. The goal of assessment is to have a better understanding of the problem to be addressed. With an understanding of health behaviors and the intrapersonal and societal forces that influence their development, maintenance, and suppression, health providers are better able to pinpoint critical factors that can serve as a basis for planning health education programs.

At this point, the planning process shifts from considering, "What is the problem?" to "What do we need to do about it?" To help in the decision as to the most appropriate type of health education program, the usual course is to assemble a planning group. The planning group should include members of the target population, or at the very least, individuals who can accurately reflect the needs of the target population, and health professionals. The planning group is responsible for developing a program plan for community health education.

Program Plan Development. Several steps are involved in developing a program plan. The first step is to identify goals for health education. Educational goals are broad statements describing what the educational intervention is being designed to accomplish. As the planning process continues, the planning group must next identify the resources and constraints that will be important in carrying out the health education program. Through this process, the planning group will develop a better sense of the likelihood of achieving the goals of education.

Defining objectives, the next step in the planning process, is perhaps the most time consuming and often frustrating activity in planning. Objectives ideally include a time frame, a specified direction of change, and how the change will be measured. In addition, to achieve success in the program, objectives must be appropriate for the target population, precise in defining the behaviors to be changed, and measurable in terms of health outcome. The planning group must select educational methods to be used in the program. The methods plus the corresponding activities provide the specifics of program operation and provide a work plan for the program.

Implementation. Depending on the scope of the program, the logistics involved with instituting plans can be overwhelming. In addition to these factors that can be anticipated, resource requirements often change through time. Planning for implementation thus becomes a difficult task. Nevertheless, developing strategies for putting the program into action is an important part of the planning process.

Program Evaluation. For program evaluation to be efficient, it should be included as an integral part of the planning process. When program planning is done carefully, the objectives developed usually provide implicit evaluation criteria. These criteria are the standards by which program achievements can be assessed. Evaluation usually takes one of two forms, process and outcome evaluation. Process evaluation is intended to determine the extent to which a program is executed so as to reach a desired goal. The actual attainment of the goal is generally not included as part of process evaluation; rather, the assumption is made that if the process is as planned, the outcome is predictable. Outcome evaluation considers the extent to which goals and objectives of a program are reached. Outcome evaluation focuses on either the impact of a program or the consequences of the impact of the program through time.

Evaluation is a necessary part of health programming. Particularly because of increased demands for accountability, evaluation is becoming more important. Evaluation is needed for monitoring the efficacy of programs, to aid in the planning of future programs, and to provide defensible evidence of the value of current programs.

In many cases, program evaluation unfortunately remains an issue that is essentially unaddressed throughout planning; it becomes a focal point only when mandated from a funding organization or other authority. When this situation occurs, program evaluation requires the use of significantly greater amounts of resources.

REFERENCES

1. Quigley, L.: The Blind Men and the Elephant: An Old Tale From the Land of India Re-Told by Lillian Quigley. New York, Scribner, 1959.
2. Squyres, W.D.: Patient Education and Health Promotion in Medical Care. Palo Alto, California, Mayfield, 1985.
3. Hochbaum, G.: Public Participation in Medical Screening Programs. Washington, USDHEW, PHS, Publication No. 572, 1958.
4. Becker, M.H., Drachman, R.H., and Kirscht, J.P.: A new approach to explaining sick-role behavior in low-income populations. Am. J. Public Health, *64*:205, 1974.
5. Rosenstock, I.M.: Historical origins of the Health Belief Model. *In* The Health Belief Model and Personal Health Behavior. Edited by M.H. Becker. Thorofare, New Jersey; Charles B. Slack, 1974.
6. McGuire, W.J.: Theoretical foundations of campaigns. *In* Public Communication Campaigns. Edited by R.E. Rice and W.J. Paisley. Beverly Hills, Sage, 1981.
7. Farquhar, J.W., Maccoby, N., and Solomon, D.S.: Community applications of behavioral medicine. *In* Handbook of Behavioral Medicine. Edited by W.D. Gentry. New York, Guilford, 1984.
8. Maccoby, N., and Solomon, D.S.: The Stanford community studies in heart disease prevention. *In* Public Communication Campaigns. Edited by R.E. Rice and W.J. Paisley. Beverly Hills, Sage, 1981.
9. Kotler, P.: Social marketing. *In* Marketing for Nonprofit Organizations. 2nd Ed. Englewood Cliffs, New Jersey, Prentice-Hall, 1982.
10. Sullivan, D.: Planning for public education about health. Washington, HEW Publication No. (HRA) 76-0074, October, 1976.
11. USDHEW, PHS, HRA: Educating the public about health: a planning guide. Washington, HEW Publication No. (HRA) 78-14004, October, 1977.
12. Warden, J.W.: Planning as a process. *In* Planning and Assessment in Community Education. Edited by H.J. Burbach and L.E. Decker. Midland, Michigan, Pendell, 1977.

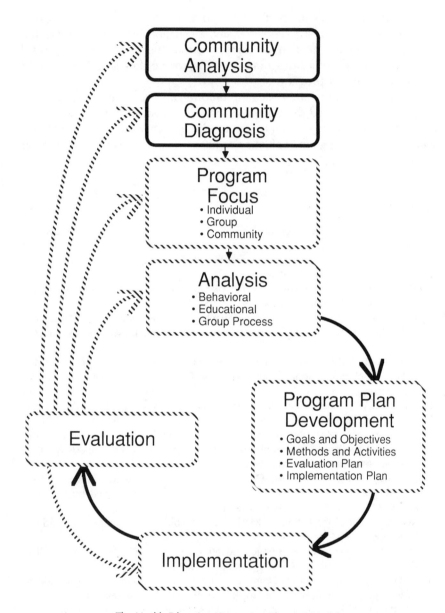

The Health Education / Promotion Planning Model.

2

Community Analysis

The most crucial elements of program planning are community analysis and diagnosis, which most health educators refer to as "needs assessment." Successful program planning in health education and health promotion depends on data gathered about the individual, group, or system that will be the focus of the program. Considering a community context for these data allows the planner to have a broad understanding of the health problem to be addressed and the resources available to address it.

Acknowledging that health education programs are most effective when they are designed for individual health problems, we must also acknowledge that individualized programs are also the least cost effective, which is a major consideration in program planning.[1] The dilemma, then, is how to plan programs that do the most for the individual and yet are within an often inadequate budget. The overall goal of an analysis of the health needs of a community is a better understanding of what makes a community function most effective. The analysis includes identification of community members; the geographic boundaries; the needs, interests, aspirations, and motivations of its members; and the effectiveness of the present health care system. Realistically, such information points to potential issues to be considered by community health educators. More detailed information is still needed before program planning can begin.

The process of community analysis often brings to light aspects of the community that heretofore have been overlooked. Community analysis provides a format whereby facts and problems pertaining to the community can be evaluated. Planners and providers can come closer to a complete understanding of the people and environment(s) to be served by identifying the needs and interests of target groups, thereby providing a basis for the development of improved services. Community analysis also provides data that are useful for identifying ineffective programs and may be used as a foundation for improvement of services through political processes. Additionally, community analysis may help individuals within the target population to understand their own problems and resources to enable them to take steps toward resolving their problems independently. When it is finished, community analysis becomes the foundation from which the need for further investigations can be identified.

UNDERSTANDING COMMUNITIES

A community may be defined by using many conceptual approaches.[2, 3] Generally speaking, "community" can be defined as functional and / or structural.

> Functional communities are nongeographic (occupational, religious, special interest, common need, or common resource) aggregates that contain the element of a place of belonging or personal identification for those involved. Structural communities are usually organized by spatial / political boundaries. They are collectives that can exist in an organizational community, such as an inpatient hospital setting; in a primary or folk community, such as a housing / apartment complex, neighborhood, parish, or ghetto; or in a legally established community called a village, town, city, county, state, or nation.[4]

The primary focus of this text is on structural communities or, as Agger states, ". . . a set of people living in a spatially bounded area that may or may not coincide with a legally bounded jurisdiction or government."[5]

Essentially, the community represents a group of individuals who share certain characteristics, such as source of income, trade center, church affiliation, or geographic location. Community members can often identify their community by name and can define the boundaries. They can identify characteristics that are shared with other members of the community and can readily identify outsiders.

Communities are made up of a variety of interactions among individuals and groups. Webber describes two basic types of interactions among community members: "place" and "non-place."[6] Place interactions are those that occur among individuals or groups within a particular geographic location, a geographic community. These are the interactions that are observed most often in our everyday activities. Non-place interactions are more subtle and often extend to locations beyond a limited geographic boundary. For example, a rural town may be defined as a community in terms of the people who rely on the goods and services available, that is, the groups of individuals who interact with the town. Thus, the community would include not only those who live within the town limits, but also those who may live outside but commonly interact with residents of the town. Identifying place interactions can be useful in understanding just what constitutes the community.

Non-place interactions may be less obvious. In our examples, even though health services may be available within the town, they may be obtained elsewhere by more isolated residents. It is common to find situations in which health care services are used for reasons other than convenience. Thus, the non-place interactions may be important to the understanding of what the concept of community means in specific situations. The concepts of place and non-place interactions are important for health educators, particularly, because patterns of interactions of clients in their own environments, away from "our" influence, often determine the success of educational programs.

The types of interactions that people have with one another and with the environment that may affect their health are numerous. When planning a program, consider the sources of information within the structural / geographic community as well as less obvious information that emerges from the study of diverse interactions within the community. Without an understanding of the nature of interactions, a complete analysis of a community is not possible.[7]

Community affiliations often provide a source of support for individuals and groups. The sense of group identity promotes motivation for change. For this reason, the community is ideal as the focal point of program planning. Program planning for a community draws upon the strengths of both individuals and groups to initiate change.

INVOLVEMENT OF HEALTH PROFESSIONALS

A health professional may be employed to begin working at any point within the cycle of program planning, program implementation, and program evaluation. Ideally, the individual would be involved in the program planning phase; however, often a proposal outlining the program has to be developed in order to acquire funds to hire staff and to initiate the program.

If the health educator becomes involved in program planning from the beginning of the administrative cycle, that is, in community analysis, he or she should utilize data that may have been gathered by other individuals, groups, or agencies. The health educator must then decide what information is needed and how it will be gathered, analyzed, and used.

FORMAT FOR COMMUNITY ANALYSIS

Various ways exist to conduct a community analysis. The format may vary from text to text, but the basic questions remain the same. A model format is presented in Table 2–1. Primarily, community analysis is an investigation of the resources and needs within a community. Through community analysis we seek to discover needs that can be fulfilled by health education programs.

Of the basic parts to a community analysis, community backdrop, analysis of the community's health status, analysis of the community's health care system, and analysis of the community's social assistance system are designed to direct information collection in areas that reflect distinct aspects of the community.[7] Community diagnosis involves the translation of the collected information into statements describing resources and needs within the community under scrutiny, and identifying target populations. Together, these parts provide information that is crucial for effective program planning.

Table 2–1. Format for Community Analysis*

		Physical and social differences in potential health-related variables
Information Collection		
Boundaries		
Backdrop		
Geographic Identifiers	Climatic	Seasonal variations in temperature and rainfall; other climatic conditions affecting health (Examples 2–1a and b)
	Surface features	Terrain, agricultural potential, natural resources (Examples 2–2a and b)
	Location	Proximity to metropolitan area; relationships to surrounding communities (Examples 2–3a and b)
Business and Commerce	Agriculture	Role in overall economy; principal cash crops; extent of agricultural development (Examples 2–4a and b)
	Industry	Extent of industrial development, types of industry, relationship between industry and the economy (Examples 2–5a and b)
	Transportation	Major means of transportation (Examples 2–6a and b)
Demographic Characteristics	Total population	Total number of residents (Examples 2–7a and b)
	Sex and age distribution	Breakdown of population into age, sex and racial characteristics (Examples 2–8a and b)
	Migration	Percent of change in population by age and sex (Examples 2–9a and b)
	Racial and ethnic groups	Percentages, by age and sex, of predominant racial and ethnic groups (Examples 2–10a and b)
	Dependency ratio	Percentage of population over 65 and under 15 years (Examples 2–11a and b)
	Family and household characteristics	Factors including housing types and conditions, single parent households, and family groups (Examples 2–12a and b)
	Educational levels	Educational levels of particular population groups (Examples 2–13a and b)
	Income and poverty	Median income by sex; extent of poverty of individuals and family groups (Examples 2–14a and b)
Social and Political Structure	Local governmental structure	Structure of local government; selection of public officials (Examples 2–15a and b)
	Educational system	Description of educational system; how leadership is selected; quality and resources within the educational system (Examples 2–16a and b)

| | Community religious practices | Predominant religious groups; relationship between religious practice and local decision making (Examples 2–17a and b) |
| | Social climate | Racial tension, labor unrest, economic struggle, political upheaval (Examples 2–18a and b) |

Community Health Status
Vital Statistics (Examples 2–19a and b)

Live birth rate	$\dfrac{\text{Number of live births}}{\text{Population of area}} \times 1000$
Fetal mortality rate	$\dfrac{\text{Number of fetal deaths}}{\text{Number of live births plus the number of fetal deaths}} \times 1000$
Infant mortality rate	$\dfrac{\text{Number of infant deaths}}{\text{Number of live births}} \times 1000$
Neonatal death rate	$\dfrac{\text{Number of neonatal deaths}}{\text{Number of live births}} \times 1000$
Death rate	$\dfrac{\text{Number of deaths}}{\text{Population of area}} \times 1000$
Causes of death	Leading causes of death by age, sex, race

Morbidity (Examples 2–20a and b)

Infectious diseases	Incidence and prevalence by age, sex, race
Noninfectious and chronic diseases	Incidence and prevalence by age, sex, race
Occupational illnesses	Incidence and prevalence by age, sex, race and duration of exposure; classified by causative agent

Community Health Care System
Manpower (Examples 2–21a and b)

Formally recognized professional groups	Sanitarians, health educators, veterinarians, nurses, nutritionists, pharmacists, medical social workers, dental hygienists, dentists, optometrists, physical therapists, occupational therapists, physicians by specialities, patient-provider ratio
Informally recognized professional groups	Folk healers, lay midwives, faith healers
Patterns of medical practice	Number of private physicians, osteopaths, dentists (Examples 2–22a and b)

Organization of Service Delivery

Colleague network among health providers	Description of local medical societies (Examples 2–23a and b)
Patient referral system	Process for finding a source of personal medical care (Examples 2–24a and b)
Hospitals	Number, location, ownership, specialty, number of beds, patient education programs (Examples 2–25a and b)

Table 2–1. Format for Community Analysis (Continued)

	Nursing homes and extended care facilities	Number, ownership, level of care (Examples 2–26a and b)
	Local health department	Basic description, organizational chart, programs (Examples 2–27a and b)
	Mental health department	Basic description, organizational structure, source of funding, level of care (Examples 2–28a and b)
	Voluntary health organizations	Lists of voluntary health organizations, recent activities (Examples 2–29a and b)
	Other rural health or inner-city health organizations	Description, sources of funds (Examples 2–30a and b)
Community's Social Assistance System Participation in Federal Programs	Medicare, Medicaid	Description of participation or non-participation (Examples 2–31a and b)
Locally Generated Programs	Local social assistance programs	Description of programs (Examples 2–32a and b)
Community Diagnosis		Determine the state of health of the community (Examples 2–33a and b)
		Determine the pattern of health services delivery in the community (Examples 2–34a and b)
		Determine the relationship between health status and health care in the community (Examples 2–35a and b)
		Identify and establish hypotheses about determinants of major problems relating to health needs and resources in the community (Examples 2–36a and b)

* Adapted from: Hochstrasser, D.L., Trapp, J.W., and Dockal, N.: Community Health Study Outline. Lexington, Kentucky, Unpublished manuscript, Department of Community Medicine, College of Medicine, Medical Center University of Kentucky, June, 1968.

The primary questions for community analysis are as follows: What questions do we ask? What are the answers? How do we interpret the answers? In addition to a proposed format for conducting a community analysis, we provide examples of the types of data readily available to those persons conducting community analyses. The examples use data available on the county level. In this discussion, Crescent County and Midland County are the communities studied. The "county" is considered the community because most data are not available at a "sub-county" level (except for large metropolitan areas).

Collecting Information

Community analysis involves collecting detailed information describing the lives of the citizens. One should begin by getting to know the area personally by inspecting and observing the community. A current map of the area is a useful tool to locate the businesses, parks, schools, hospitals, physicians' offices, and public health department and other governmental services. Other ways to learn about the community include driving through neighborhoods or other places where people live, observing predominant housing types, learning the geographic layout of the housing patterns within the community, meeting with merchants and community residents to learn about their daily routines, reading newspapers and other local printed media, listening to local radio, and watching locally produced television programs. Notes should be kept and questions should be answered before any further analysis is done.

Defining Boundaries

After an initial inspection, tentative boundaries of the community should be defined. These boundaries are important, because they may be used to define target areas for future programs. Boundaries should reflect major differences in potential health-related variables such as housing, accessibility to services, predominant racial makeup, or school districts. Obvious choices are major physical boundaries such as rivers or major streets, governmental boundaries such as school districts, and city limits.[8] Special attention must be given to avoid choosing boundaries simply for convenience; rather, the boundaries should serve to delimit discrete sections of the community. Such boundaries may be drawn along lines reflecting housing type, employment, de facto racial segregation, or predominant age of residents. The mythical Crescent and Midland Counties serve as examples.

Crescent County is bordered on the west by the Crescent River. The largest city within the county, Rapid City, developed as a commercial center along the railway system that runs through the heart of the county, north to south. The population of Rapid City is 28,160.

Numerous rural communities exist throughout the county that appear to focus around a neighborhood church, a community store, and a school or recreation center. Several of the communities have a volunteer rescue squad and fire department.

In addition to Rapid City, there is only one other incorporated city, Oak Grove, which is located in the southeast corner of the county. The population of Oak Grove is about 9,280.

Crescent County, Rapid City, and Oak Grove are recognized as formal governmental units. The boundaries of the county are firmly established; however, the boundaries of the cities are subject to change upon additional annexation. The boundaries of the rural communities cannot be established until more extensive community analysis is carried out with local residents.

Midland County is heavily developed and the population density is high.[9, 10] It is a leading trade center for the region.

Numerous municipalities are located in Midland County. Metrocity is the largest urban area and is the county seat. Suburban growth is rapid and expansive.

Backdrop

Community analysis also involves defining the backdrop of the community. The backdrop is analogous to the scenery in a play; it contributes to the mood and provides the environment within which the characters function and the plot develops. The information collected as the backdrop of the community helps to describe the relevant characteristics of the setting that in turn reveal health aspects of the area. Primary descriptors of the community backdrop include geographic identifiers, business and commerce, demographic characteristics, and social and political structures.

Geographic Identifiers. These include climate, surface features, and location. Considerations related to *climate* are seasonal variations in temperature and rainfall, as well as any other climatic conditions that may affect the health of community residents.

> Example 2–1a. Crescent County has an altitude of 600 feet above sea level. The climate is temperate, with a mean temperature of 62.7°F. The average annual rainfall is 48 inches. Summers are hot and humid. Winters are cold but with little snow; average annual snowfall is 6 inches.

> Example 2–1b. Midland County has an elevation of 550 feet above sea level. The mean temperature in January is 28°F and in July, 78°F. The average monthly amount of precipitation is 2.1 inches. Four distinct seasons exist, with a growing season of about 170 days; snow cover exists about 60 days of the year.

Surface features include the terrain, agricultural potential, and natural resources of the area.

> Example 2–2a. Crescent County has a gently rolling terrain. The soil is rocky and composed mostly of clay. The dominant surface feature in the county is the Crescent River, a broad, shallow river typical of others in the central part of the state. The river forms the western boundary of the county.
>
> The wooded areas are predominantly hardwood—oaks and poplars—interspersed with pines and cedars. The northwest area of the county is more wooded and geographically isolated than any other part of the county. There is some timbering currently underway in this area.

Example 2–2b. Midland County is noted for rolling farmland crossed by dense hardwood forests and three major rivers. The bays and rivers are amenable to navigation. The characteristics of local soil make it suitable for agriculture.

Location reveals proximity to metropolitan areas (if rural) and relationship to surrounding communities.

Example 2–3a. Crescent County is located in the central area of the state. To the west of Crescent County, the land becomes mountainous. Toward the east, the land flattens into the coastal plain.

Crescent County is in an excellent location for industrial and commercial growth. An interstate highway and railroad system that crosses the county promotes interstate and intrastate trade.

Example 2–3b. Metrocity is the largest urban area in Midland County. Three other urban areas within the county have a population of over 25,000. Six additional cities within a 100-mile radius have a population of over 100,000. These areas of high population density are interconnected by major highways and other modes of transportation.

Business and Commerce. Business and commerce are described through study of the agriculture, industry, and transportation of the community. The importance of *agriculture* to the overall economy, principal cash crops, and the extent of agricultural development throughout the county should be identified. Information regarding the agricultural history of the area will help to explain the economic background of the area.

Example 2–4a. About 48% of the population of Crescent County (72,000) lives in rural areas—40% in areas considered rural non-farm and 8% in areas considered rural farm. Until about 40 years ago, the major source of income was farming.

Much of the county has been timbered, providing open farmland and pastures. Most of the farmland is planted in grains, corn, and soybeans. The pasture areas support both dairy and beef cattle.

Example 2–4b. Agriculture and supporting businesses are the second largest source of income for Midland County. Principal cash crops and agricultural products include soybeans, corn, grain, and livestock. Most farming takes place on commercial farms that comprise at least 300 acres. The extent of rapid urban and suburban growth is decreasing the amount of land available for agricultural use.

Industry studies explain the extent of industrial development, the types of industry, and the relationship between industry and the economy.

Example 2–5a. Of all employed persons, 54% are employed in manufacturing industries. These industries are mainly hosiery, fabric-weaving, and garment sewing textile companies. In addition, a growing number of industries manufacture durable goods.

There is an adequate pool of local manpower to support the current industrial growth. Industries constantly seek to move into Crescent County because of the labor pool, natural resources, and access to industrial highways and the railroad.

Since industries began moving into Crescent County about 30 to 40 years ago, there has been a steady change in employment patterns. Both women and men are now employed in the industrial sector, displacing the primary source of income from the family farm to the factory.

Example 2–5b. Industrial development is extensive. In addition to agriculture-related industries, the manufacture of steel, machinery, and other types of durable goods lead this development. Chemical industries continue to expand. The geographic location of Midland County and the expansive transportation system continue to make Metrocity a rapidly growing urban center with an expanding economy.

Industrial development is heaviest on the southeast side of Metrocity and along the rivers and bays. Industries are following the population movement into suburban areas.

Table 2-2.   Sex, Age, and Race Distribution in Crescent County

		All Races		White		Non-white	
	Total	Male	Female	Male	Female	Male	Female
All ages	72,000	34,560	37,440	28,800	31,680	5,040	6,480
<5	5,760	2,736	3,024	2,095	2,268	641	756
5-14	14,400	7,344	7,056	5,760	5,400	1,584	1,656
15-19	7,200	3,960	3,240	2,844	2,772	792	792
20-64	38,880	18,216	20,664	15,869	18,576	1,663	2,772
65+	5,760	2,304	3,456	2,232	2,664	360	504

Transportation identification specifies major means of transportation for daily use and for travel out of the immediate area. Highway, air, and marine or river transportation systems are included.

> Example 2-6a. No locally operated public transportation systems exist within Crescent County. There are two local taxi companies based in Rapid City. The railroad and commercial bus lines provide intercity transportation.
> Transportation for special groups is available to a limited extent. For example, the Council on Aging, the Urban Development Center, and the county Recreation Department has vans and cars to transport their clients. Thirteen percent of all housing units have no automobile.
> Commercial transportation routes are enhanced by a Regional Airport located 30 miles from Rapid City in James County, the next county to the east.

> Example 2-6b. Transportation networks are extensive. Major interstate highways cross the area. Four major railroad systems, two airlines, and four transit systems serve Metrocity. The three navigable rivers also support the shipping industry.

Demographic Characteristics. These include total population, sex and age distribution, migration, racial and ethnic groups, dependency ratio, family and household characteristics, educational levels, and income and poverty. Total population is the total number of residents residing within the area.

> Example 2-7a. The total population of Crescent County is 72,000 residents.

> Example 2-7b. The population of Metrocity is 1,000,000; the total population of Midland County is 1,500,000.[10] Of the population of Midland County, 81% live in urban areas. Suburban growth has increased 40% in the past 10 years. Midland County has a higher percentage of residents employed in manufacturing, transportation, wholesale / retail, finance, and service areas than does the United States as a whole. The percentage of workers employed in the fields of construction and government service in Midland County is lower than the national percentages in these categories.

Sex and age distribution include a breakdown of the population into age, sex, and racial characteristics.

> Example 2-8a. (See Table 2-2).
> Example 2-8b. (See Table 2-3.)

Migration describes the percent of change in the population, by age and sex, over the past decade.

> Example 2-9a. An approximate 8% in-migration has occurred for Crescent County within the last 10 years. The rate of in-migration appears to parallel the industrial growth in the county. Rapid City is growing more quickly than the rest of the county and is the area where most new residents settle. Many of the newcomers represent the 35 to 50-year-old male, managerial, manpower that have moved into the county with new industries. Approximately 15% of employed persons in Crescent County work outside the county.

Table 2–3. Sex, Age, and Race Distribution in Midland County

Ages	All Races		White		Black		Spanish and Other Origin	
	Male	Female	Male	Female	Male	Female	Male	Female
	718,500	781,500	476,640	516,360	166,980	196,020	74,880	69,120
<5	54,606	53,142	29,075	27,883	17,199	17,053	8,332	8,206
5–9	55,324	53,142	29,552	28,399	18,033	18,034	7,739	6,709
10–14	60,354	58,613	35,271	33,563	18,368	18,622	6,715	6,428
15–19	68,258	67,209	41,468	40,276	19,369	20,190	7,421	6,743
18+	506,543	575,966	357,003	401,728	101,189	129,961	48,351	44,277
65+	63,228	100,032	51,000	82,101	9,685	14,309	2,543	3,622

Example 2–9b. Migration into Midland County is steady. A similarly steady movement into suburban areas is represented by an increase in suburban population of 40% in the past 10 years. Recent in-migration has been from other states. Most new residents are young adults seeking employment in the city.

Racial and ethnic groups are identified by percentages of age and sex of predominant racial and ethnic groups.

Example 2–10a. Approximately 12% of the population of Crescent County is black and 4% is composed of Japanese, Chinese, Filipinos, and other groups. Specific age and sex categories are given in Example 2–8a, Table 2–2.

Example 2–10b. Midland County has a population that is 66.2% white, 24.2% black, and 9.6% of Spanish and other origins. Metrocity has numerous distinct ethnic neighborhoods. These neighborhoods include persons of German, Italian, Polish, and Irish descent.

Dependency ratio is the ratio of the sum of the population over 65 years plus those under 15 years divided by the total population.[11]

Example 2–11a. In Crescent County, 5760 residents are over the age of 65 years—8% of the total population. There are 20,160 children under the age of 15 years—28% of the population. Thus the dependency ratio is 25,920 to 72,000, or approximately 1:2.8. By comparison, 9% of the state's population is over 65 years and 30% is under the age of 15 years.

Example 2–11b. In Midland County, 7.2% of the population is under 5 years of age, 26.4% is 5 to 14 years of age, 9.0% is 15 to 19 years of age, and 10.9% is over 65 years of age. Of the total population, 72.2% is over 18 years of age.

Family and household characteristics include many factors that may require study. These factors may include housing types and conditions (percent substandard), single-parent households, family groups, and any other patterns of lifestyle encountered.

Example 2–12a. Approximately 19,940 families live in Crescent County, with 10,800 of these families having children of their own under 18 years of age. Although there are about the same number of men and women in the county—34,560 and 37,440, respectively—approximately six times as many women are widowed and twice as many are divorced. There are 1728 families that are headed by a woman. Five percent of the households are single-parent households.

In Crescent County there are 3.2 persons per housing unit. Eleven percent of the housing units lack some or all plumbing facilities. Most of the rural farm and non-farm homes are of wood frame construction. Within the last 10 years, building in the rural areas has increased. Most new construction has helped to increase the availability of adequate housing.

Example 2–12b. The large urban area is marked by concentrated housing. The percentage of women in the labor force in Midland County is higher than in the country as a whole.

Statistics show 77.4% of the men over 16 years of age are in the labor force and 53.5% of the women over 16 years of age are in the labor force. The divorce rate (per 1000) is 4.5 and the marriage rate (per 1000) is 9.0.

Educational levels determine the educational levels of particular population groups. This determination is especially valuable as a basis of planning health education programs.

Example 2–13a. In Crescent County, the median of school years completed for persons 25 years and older is 10.1, as compared to 10.9 for the state. More detailed statistics on educational levels are not readily available.

Example 2–13b. In Midland County, 65.2% of the population 25 years of age and older have completed 4 years of high school and 15.8% have completed at least 4 years of college.

Income and poverty concerns are identified by the median income by sex and the extent of poverty of individuals and family groups.

Example 2–14a. In Crescent County, 2.6% of the work force is unemployed as compared to 3.2% for the state. Sixty percent of women ages 15 to 44 years in Crescent County are employed. The mean family income is $9700; for female-headed families, the mean income is $6000.

Of Crescent County families, 9.5% have incomes less than the poverty level, as compared to 14% for the state.

Of Crescent County families, 10.1% receive public assistance or public welfare income.

Example 2–14b. The per capita annual income in Midland County is $7904. Of families in Midland County, 9.8% have incomes below the poverty level; 9.9% of these households receive some form of public assistance. The number of residents needing special support services is increasing, but the local tax base is decreasing. The percentage of residents in Midland County who are unemployed is higher than for the country as a whole.

Social and Political Structure. This information is revealed through study of local government structure, educational systems, community religious practices, and social climate. *Local governmental structure* describes the structure of local government and the selection of public officials.

Example 2–15a. Crescent County is governed by a Board of County Commissioners. A county manager is employed by the county. The human service agencies operate as separate entities.

There is a city-county planning office in which a human services planner has been employed for the last 5 years. This individual works with all human service agencies in the county to assist in planning budgets, programs, and expansions, and especially serves as an advocate for continuity of care from all county agencies.

All county agencies are governed by boards appointed by the county commissioners. The local Board of Health meets monthly with the health department's management staff. This Board has become more involved and concerned with preventive health issues within Crescent County.

Example 2–15b. Metrocity is the county seat of Midland County. Numerous city, county, state, and federal government offices are located in Metrocity.

Educational system assessments may be helpful in determining the quality of and resources within the educational system.

Example 2–16a. Crescent County has two public school systems, the Crescent County Schools and the Rapid City Schools. Few children in the county attend private schools. The teacher to pupil ratio is 1:30.

Within the county schools, a committee was established to work with the curriculum director on health and science courses. The committee has met once in the last 6 months.

In Crescent County Technical Institute, a growing number of human service preparation courses are taught. In addition, Crescent County has Braxton College; which is supported by the Baptist Church and has a student body of 2800.

Example 2–16b. Midland County has three major universities and two major medical centers.

One third of the elementary and secondary schools and three fifths of the institutions of higher education are private.

Community religious practices reveal predominant religious groups, by economic strata and racial or ethnic characteristics. The extent of religious practice, especially as related to the local decision-making process, should be investigated.

Example 2–17a. Baptists, Methodists, and Presbyterians represent the predominant religious groups within Crescent County. Religious identity in the county is strong. The church often serves as the focus of community activity. Most of the county officials are equally active in church functions.

Most public officials, board members, and community leaders are members of churches within the county. Although community leaders do not use the church as a public forum, their stands on particular issues often reflect those of their church.

Several churches have become more involved with community health projects within the last few years. Some issues addressed included isolation and care of the elderly, adolescent health, and family unity.

Example 2–17b. The predominant religious groups include Catholic, Lutheran, Methodist, Presbyterian, Episcopalian, and Unitarian denominations. There is also a large Jewish population in Midland County.

Social climate includes a description and explanation of racial tension, labor unrest, economic struggle, and political upheaval.

Example 2–18a. There appears to be little social strife within Crescent County. The most tense event recalled by residents involved a labor strike at the largest local textile mill in 1974. This strike drew public attention to work conditions and wages, resulting in both the layoff of a number of workers and some increase in wages and health benefits.

Crescent County is a growing and prosperous county. There are numerous social organizations that sponsor community development and community service projects. There is a growing population of senior citizens who have difficulty maintaining households on fixed incomes.

Example 2–18b. Several major events of social and economic unrest have occurred within Metrocity. Unemployment and other economic issues were their basic cause. The crime rate in Midland County is 5283 crimes per 100,000 residents.

Using the information collected we now have useful descriptors for a comprehensive backdrop. We can now identify the community as well as its related countryside, sources of influence or power upon the community, major social groups including racial or ethnic groups and migrants, social stratification, power structures that dominate the community, and the extent of conflict and / or cooperation among various groups and forces within the community. These community descriptors provide a good "backdrop." As we learn more about health-related concerns and issues within the community, they can be incorporated into the backdrop, and perhaps provide useful insight into complex problems.

Analysis of Community Health Status

Collection of relevant data describing the health status of the population in the community is the next part of the community analysis. These data, when synthesized, are useful in determining the most pressing health needs of the community.

Perhaps the most basic data useful in determining community health status are vital statistics and morbidity data. Vital statistics should include data collected for the previous decade and be compared to state and national statistics. Pay attention to units determining rates. A rate of 5 per 100,000 is not the same as 5 per 1000.

Vital Statistics

Live Birth Rate. "Live birth is the complete expulsion or extraction from its mother of a product of conception, irrespective of the duration of pregnancy, which, after separation, breathes or shows any other evidence of life, such as beating of the heart, pulsation of the umbilical cord, or any definite movement of voluntary muscles, whether or not the umbilical cord has been cut or the placenta is attached."[12]

$$\text{Birth rate} = \frac{\text{number of live births}}{\text{population of area}} \times 1000$$

Example 2–19a. Live birth rate.
State: 14.9 per 1000 population
Crescent County: 12.7 per 1000 population
Midland County: 15.8 per 1000 population

Fetal Mortality Rate. "Fetal death is death prior to the complete expulsion or extraction from its mother of a product of human conception, irrespective of the duration of pregnancy, as indicated by the fact that after such expulsion or extraction the fetus does not breathe or show any evidence of life, such as beating of the heart, pulsation of the umbilical cord, or definite movement of voluntary muscles."[12]

$$\text{Fetal mortality rate} = \frac{\text{number of fetal deaths}}{\substack{\text{number of live births plus} \\ \text{the number of fetal deaths}}} \times 1000$$

Example 2–19a, continued. Fetal mortality rate.
State: 11.0 per 1000 deliveries
Crescent County: 10.8 per 1000 deliveries
Midland County: 11.2 per 1000 deliveries

Infant Mortality Rate. "Infant death is defined as death of a liveborn infant under 1 year of age."[12]

$$\text{Infant mortality rate} = \frac{\text{number of infant deaths}}{\text{number of live births}} \times 1000$$

Example 2–19a, continued. Infant mortality rate.
State: 12.8 per 1000 live births

Table 2–4. Leading Causes of Death in Crescent County*

	State	Crescent County
Infective and parasitic diseases	10.3	12.1
Neoplasms	164.9	182.3
Diabetes mellitus	14.5	11.7
Endocrine, nutritional, and metabolic diseases	18.2	23.4
Mental disorders	9.7	7.2
Diseases of the nervous system and sense organs	8.8	6.9
Diseases of the circulatory system	434.8	442.5
Diseases of the respiratory system	54.2	50.1
Diseases of the digestive system	27.9	14.8
Diseases of the genitourinary system	14.1	11.7
Diseases of the musculoskeletal system	1.3	1.1
Congenital anomalies	6.4	5.8
Certain causes of mortality in early infancy	12.1	10.8
Accidents, poisonings, and violence (all causes)	82.5	74.3

* Rate by cause per 100,000 population.

Crescent County: 11.4 per 1000 live births
Midland County: 13.9 per 1000 live births

Neonatal Death Rate. "Neonatal death is death of a liveborn child under 28 days of age."[12]

$$\text{Neonatal death rate} = \frac{\text{number of neonatal deaths}}{\text{number of live births}} \times 1000$$

Example 2–19a, continued. Neonatal death rate.
State: 9.1 per 1000 neonatal survivors
Crescent County: 7.4 per 1000 neonatal survivors
Midland County: 7.9 per 1000 neonatal survivors

Death Rate.

$$\text{Death rate} = \frac{\text{number of deaths}}{\text{population of area}} \times 1000$$

Example 2–19a, continued. Death rate.
State: 8.1 per 1000 population
Crescent County: 8.6 per 1000 population
Midland County: 8.9 per 1000 population

Causes of Death. Indicate leading causes of death by age, sex, and race (age ranges should begin under 1 year of age, 1–4, 5–14, 15–24 ... 65–74, 75+). If the causes of death are identified according to age, sex, and race, particular groups in need or who experience unusually high death rates can be identified.

Example 2–19a, continued. In Crescent County, most deaths from infective and parasitic diseases occur in Caucasian women over 55 years of age. Neoplasia is a significant cause of death to Crescent County residents over 45 years of age, with slightly higher rates noted for Caucasians than for non-Caucasians, and for male than for female residents. Death from endocrine, nutritional, and metabolic diseases occurs primarily in residents over the age of 55 years. More men than women and more non-Caucasian than Caucasian persons are affected. Death related to diseases of the circulatory system occurs primarily in residents over the age of 45 years. Men are affected more often than are women and Caucasians more often than non-Caucasians.

Example 2–19b.

Table 2–5.   Leading Causes of Death in Midland County*

	State	Midland County
Heart disease	326.0	359.2
Malignant neoplasia	195.8	201.7
Cerebrovascular disease	67.9	68.0
Accidents	31.9	32.8
COPD †	22.8	25.1
Pneumonia and influenza	21.4	22.7
Diabetes	15.3	18.4
Suicide	12.5	9.8
Chronic liver disease and cirrhosis	11.9	12.8
Atherosclerosis	11.0	11.5
Homicide	10.4	14.2

* Rate by cause per 100,000 population.
† Chronic obstructive pulmonary disease.

Morbidity Data. Morbidity data reveal the most common illnesses in the community. Comparison of local rates with state, regional, or national data is often indicative of the effectiveness of preventive health programs. The following data are needed.

Infectious Diseases. It is important to know the incidence and prevalence of infectious diseases by age, sex, and race within a community to help isolate particular health problems and affected populations.

> Example 2–20a. Communicable disease morbidity data are not available by age, sex, and race for Crescent County. Problems with securing accurate reporting mechanisms as well as the small numbers of cases of particular diseases present problems in interpretation of the data.
>
> Example 2–20b. Selected morbidity rates (per 1000 residents) for Midland County are: gonorrhea, 485.7; syphilis, 35.2; hepatitis, 30.4; and tuberculosis, 29.9. Rates for gonorrhea, hepatitis, and tuberculosis are higher than the national average.

Noninfectious and Chronic Diseases. Indicate incidence and prevalence by age, sex, race, and occupation. Many of the noninfectious and chronic diseases have causative factors that can be regulated by individual health behavior. Various health education programs play an important role in informing the general public regarding these diseases as well as educating groups and individuals on measures to help alleviate or stabilize the problem.

As with infectious diseases, data on noninfectious and chronic diseases by age, sex, and race help pinpoint populations with a higher concentration, or for comparative purposes, a lower concentration, of problems.

> Example 2–20a, continued. Although there are no current data on the exact numbers of individuals in Crescent County who have certain noninfectious and chronic diseases, approximations are given in Table 2–7.
>
> Additional morbidity data could be gathered from the two local hospitals, clinics, private industries, and perhaps the Grandview Health Systems Agency.

Occupational Illnesses. Data on incidence and prevalence by age, sex, race, and duration of exposure are seldom available. Occupational diseases result from the inhalation, ingestion, or contact with the skin of toxic and irritating substances.[15] The substances or hazards resulting in occupational

Table 2–6. Incidence of Infectious Diseases per 100,000 Population in Crescent County

	State	Crescent County
Amebiasis	0.18	0.0
Encephalitis	0.85	1.0
Hepatitis A and unspecified	7.86	6.0
Measles (rubeola)	2.02	0.0
Mumps	1.54	1.0
Rocky Mountain spotted fever	3.81	12.0
German measles (rubella)	5.05	41.0
Salmonellosis	16.10	13.0
Shigellosis	3.38	2.0
Tetanus	0.13	0.0
Tuberculosis (all forms)	17.87	10.0
Typhoid fever	0.07	0.0
Whooping cough	1.05	1.0
Venereal diseases		
Gonorrhea (genitourinary)	690.62	689.0
Syphilis (all stages)	33.45	28.0
Chancroid	0.02	0.0
Nonspecific urethritis	67.56	35.0

illnesses may be biologic hazards, dermatoses, substances affecting the airways and lungs, plant and wood hazards, chemical hazards, chemical carcinogens, pesticides, or physical hazards. Occupational illnesses are often classified according to the causative agent.[15] Data from the worksite may

Table 2–7. Approximate Numbers of Individuals with Infectious and Chronic Diseases in Crescent County

Hypertension	
Population over 18 years	44,640
Population with hypertension (23.2% of the population over 18 years)	10,356
Glaucoma	
Population over 35 years	31,401
Population with glaucoma (2% of the population over 35 years)	628
Epilepsy	
Total population	72,000
Population with epilepsy (1% of the population)	720
In need of Home Health Services	
0.5% of the population under 65 years	331
10% of the population over 65 years	576
Total estimated population in need of home health services	907
Cervical Cancer	
Number of women 20 years of age and older	24,120
Expected new cases of cervical cancer 0.0009 of women over 20 years)	22
Breast Cancer	
Number of women 20 years of age and older	24,120
Expected new cases of breast cancer 0.0013 of women over 20 years)	31

(From U.S. Bureau of the Census: Statistical Abstract of the United States, 1986. 106th Ed. Washington, 1985; American Heart Association: Heart Facts. Dallas, 1985; State of North Carolina, Department of Human Resources, Division of Health Services: Memorandum to Local Health Directors from W.B. Jones, M.D., regarding chronic disease program planning workshops. Raleigh, January 27, 1978.)

Table 2–8.   Annual Work-Related Injuries, by Industry, Crescent County

Total cases	932	Wholesale Trade	27
Agriculture	5	Retail Trade	81
Mining	1	Finance	4
Construction	96	Service	78
Manufacturing	568	Public Administration	30
Transportation, etc.	42		

include information regarding employee absenteeism rates, accident rates, and insurance claims. Health promotion and health education programs are often based on these data.

Example 2–20a, continued. In Crescent County, work-related fatalities occur most often in manufacturing, construction, transportation, public utilities, and public administration occupations.

The most common types of work-related injuries are strains, sprains, fractures, cuts, punctures, and bruises. Occupational accidents most often affect the back, fingers, and legs.

In Crescent County, 932 work accidents were recorded during the year. Two of these accidents resulted in fatalities and 536 were disabling.

Work-related injuries for particular industries in Crescent County during the year are presented in Table 2–8. More work-related injuries occur in manufacturing industries than in any other industry. Almost one third of all the manufacturing industry injuries occurred in textile mill and apparel products. These injuries can be described as primarily chemical burns, dermatitis and inflammation, or irritation of the joints. Data on these injuries and other occupational health hazards are not readily available for Crescent County.

Example 2–20b. Concern for the occupational health of Midland County workers has increased as more informaton is gained about unhealthy conditions. The manufacturing industries constitute the largest category of employment, and also have the greatest number of occupational work-related accidents.

The number of health promotion and work safety programs within the worksites in Midland County is increasing. These programs along with OSHA regulations and union involvement have increased the attention placed on the workers and work environment issues.

These data help to clarify what experiences make a community's health patterns unique. Are there any striking differences between statistics of death and illness among the community, the state, or the nation as a whole? Are any trends evident? What age, sex, or racial groups experience the most or the least premature death?

Analysis of the Community Health Care System

The subsequent part of the community analysis is designed to collect and synthesize data describing the resources for providing health care in the community. If a community is even marginally isolated, many residents may rely on other communities for health care. To know which community services are being used by the residents, it may be necessary to conduct a survey of a sample of the citizens. More likely, data are available from the state health planning agencies. In any event, obtain information concerning the availability of manpower and the organization of service delivery for the health care system in a community.

Table 2–9. Numbers of Practicing Health Care Professionals in Crescent County

Sanitarians		5	Physicians by specialty:	
Health educators		1	Allergy	1
Veterinarians		12	Dermatology	2
Nurses	215 RNs	160 LPNs	Family practice	12
Nutritionists		3	General practice	8
Pharmacists		20	Gynecology and obstetrics	8
Medical social workers		58	Internal medicine	8
Dentists		40	Neurology	7
Optometrists		12	Ophthalmology	3
Physical therapists		5	Orthopedics	6
Occupational therapists		4	Otorhinolaryngology	4
Total number of health			Pediatrics	8
care professionals		535	Psychiatry	1
			Surgery	7
			Other	3
			Total number of physicians	78

Availability of Manpower. The availability of manpower can be assessed through the following research.

Formally Recognized Professional Groups. Indicate the numbers of practicing sanitarians, health educators, veterinarians, nurses, nutritionists, pharmacists, medical social workers, dental hygienists, dentists, optometrists, physical therapists, occupational therapists, and physicians by specialty. Determine the patient-provider ratio. The physician to population ratio for Crescent County is 1 to 923, as compared with a ratio of 1 to 789 for the state (see Table 2–9).

Example 2–21a. Most of the physicians in Crescent County are based in Rapid City around the two hospitals. Several physicians are located in Oak Grove. Other than those located in Oak Grove, there are no physicians in the more rural areas.

Example 2–21b. Most of the major professional groups have a county or state-level professional organization. Within Midland County, there are numerous councils staffed by professionals. The purpose of these councils is for information sharing and problem solving.

Informally Recognized Practitioners. Indicate numbers of "folk" healers, lay midwives, faith healers, "quacks," and others.

Example 2–21a, continued. Even though it is impossible to document the exact number of folk healers in Crescent County, there are two types of informally recognized practitioners within the county, faith healers and herbalists. Senior citizens and young adults utilize these practitioners more than other county residents.

Areas Identified as Medically Underserved. Medically underserved areas may be identified according to accessibility as well as by patient-provider ratio.

Example 2–21a, continued. Most of the health and medical manpower are based within Rapid City. There are several physicians in Oak Grove. Because the interstate highway runs east to west through the midst of the county, and the river forms a natural barrier on the west, the northwest area of the county is considered medically underserved. Transportation time to Rapid City from Bryson's Fork, a northwest community, is 30 minutes in good weather. There are no physicians in that area of the county. In addition, county agencies can provide only limited coverage to that area.

In contrast to being underserved because of geographic isolation, several older communities south of the interstate that are within a few miles of Rapid City limits have demonstrated hardship in reaching medical services. Local ambulance services report a high rate of calls from these areas; however, often these individuals only need transportation to a medical facility.

Example 2–21b, continued. Several isolated inner-city neighborhoods are considered medically underserved. Over the past 15 years, federally funded projects have been directed toward these communities.

Organization of Service Delivery. The organization of service delivery can be investigated in the following manner.

Pattern of Medical Practice. Indicate the number of private physicians, osteopaths, dentists, and other practitioners. (Make note if patient education is emphasized in any of these practices.)

Example 2–22a. About one half of all physicians in the county have solo practices. There is a trend toward small group practices, especially among physicians with specialty practices. Most of the larger group practices are located near the county's privately owned hospital, Crescent Memorial Hospital. There are no prepaid group practices such as health maintenance organizations within the county.

Example 2–22b. There are 74 non-resident primary care physicians, 25 physician assistants, 282 licensed practical nurses, and 604 registered nurses per 100,000 Midland County residents.

Colleague Network. Describe this association among health providers, i.e., local medical societies.

Example 2–23a. A county medical society meets monthly, except during the summer. The medical society has social, political, professional, and educational functions. Approximately every other month, the program is of an educational nature. Most programs focus on new governmental regulations pertaining to Medicaid, Medicare, hospital care or expansion, and current trends in medical care. The county medical society has delegates to the state medical society.

Example 2–23b. There is a city-based medical society. Most practitioners' associations are sponsored through the Midland County hospital and medical centers. These groups focus their efforts on cost containment, alternative forms of medical care, and program administration.

Patient Referral System. Describe how people in the community find a source of health care when needed.

Example 2–24a. Even though most long-time Crescent County residents state that they have no trouble securing medical care, many newcomers express difficulty in finding a family physician. Emergency room personnel at the local hospital report that they see many individuals with non-crisis complaints who could be seen by a general practitioner.

The increase in the number of physicians in the county has been in specialized practices. Local agencies and the local medical society refer newcomers to physicians and specialists as needed and requested.

Example 2–24b. The Midland County Hospital System provides care to indigent residents.

Hospital(s). Specify the number, location, type of ownership, speciality, and number of beds in area hospitals. Indicate if patient education is included.

Example 2–25a. The two hospitals in Crescent County are Crescent Memorial and Crescent County General Hospital. Crescent Memorial Hospital operates as a private nonprofit hospital, whereas Crescent County Hospital is publicly supported. Both hospitals are located in Rapid City and are within four miles of each other.

Neither hospital has a formalized patient education program. Patient education within the hospitals is on an individual patient basis and is conducted by the nurses and physicians.

Both the chaplain and the Patient Concerns Representative from Memorial Hospital have expressed interest in developing patient education programs.

Example 2–25b. There are two major medical centers and 24 public and private hospitals in Midland County, providing 72.4 hospital beds per 1000 residents. The occupancy rate for hospitals in Midland County is 74.1.

Nursing Homes and Extended Care Facilities. Specify the number, ownership, and level of care certification for nursing homes and extended care facilities.

Example 2–26a. In Crescent County, nursing homes and extended care facilities include skilled nursing homes, intermediate care facilities, homes for the aged, and family care units. Skilled nursing homes include 24-hour nursing coverage and have a registered nurse as Director of Nursing. Intermediate care facilities, depending upon their level of certification, may or may not have nursing coverage. Homes for the aged do not require nursing coverage for licensure. Family care units are similar to homes for the aged with the exception that they are licensed for only five or fewer individuals.

In Crescent County, three facilities provide both skilled nursing services and intermediate care services. These facilities are licensed for 93 skilled nursing beds and 114 intermediate care beds. About 60% of nursing home patients who go to Crescent County nursing homes are from Crescent County. There are four homes for the aged that are licensed for a total of 146 beds. In addition, there are 10 family care units in Crescent County licensed for a total of 40 beds.

Most of the nursing homes and extended care facilities in Crescent County are privately owned. Several of the facilities are private, nonprofit church-related facilities.

Example 2–26b. All levels of care (residential, intermediate, multilevel, and skilled nursing) are available in nursing homes in Midland County. The services provided are primarily domiciliary, nursing, and personal care. The number of skilled nursing and intermediate care facilities has shown steady growth.

The nursing homes are categorized as public, nonprofit, or proprietary. There are 72 skilled nursing and intermediate facilities in Midland County, with a 98.1 occupancy rate in these facilities.

Local Health Department. Describe the local health department, indicating whether it is city, county, or regionally governed. Include the legal authority of the department in this description.

Example 2–27a. The county health department is located on the southeast side of Rapid City. There is one health department-sponsored outreach or community clinic based in Oak Grove.

The building that houses the health department was constructed as a specialty hospital in 1947 and operated as such until 11 years ago. At that time, the county health department moved into the facility.

The health department has a staff of about 75 employees.

Example 2–27b. The health department in Midland County is staffed by 1500 full-time employees and is governed by an Advisory Council. The department is organized into four major units, the Bureau of Environmental Health, the Bureau of Supporting Services, the Bureau of Community Health Services and the Bureau of Personal Health Services. Health education is under the auspices of the Bureau of Community Health Services.

Obtain an *organizational chart* for the local health department that, at a minimum, identifies key decision-makers. Indicate where health education is within the organization and describe its functions. A sample chart for Crescent County is provided in Figure 2–1.

List the *programs,* such as immunizations, family planning, and clinics, provided by the health department.

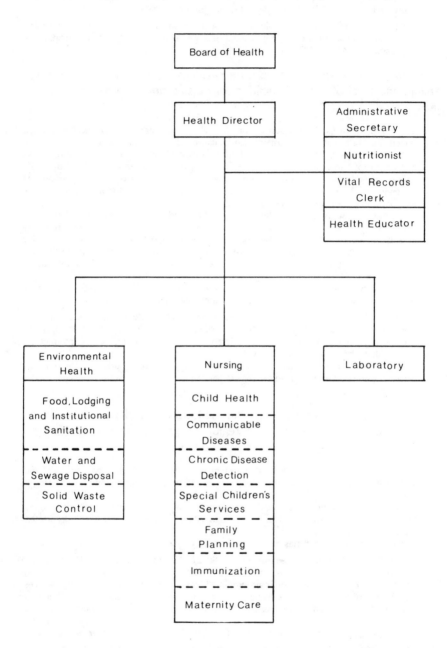

Fig. 2-1. Organizational chart of the Crescent County Health Department.

Example 2–27a, continued. The Crescent County Health Department-sponsored clinically based programs include child health, chronic disease detection, communicable disease (such as venereal disease and tuberculosis), special children's services, family planning, immunization, maternity care, and health promotion. All of these programs have an outreach or community health component. Nurses, outreach workers, and other program staff make home visits and work with community groups to foster these programs.

The health educator and nutritionist work within the clinically based programs to provide patient education. Their community contact is limited and is on a "request" basis.

The health department also undertakes sizable environmental health programs. These include food, lodging, and institutional sanitation; water and sewage disposal; and solid waste control. These programs are predominantly community based.

In addition to clinically based and community-based programs, there are support services such as the laboratory and vital records within the health department.

Example 2–27b, continued. The categorical programs within the health department in Metrocity include dental care; maternity; Women, Infants, and Children (WIC); home health; sexually transmitted diseases; communicable disease control; school health; Early, Periodic, Screening and Diagnosis and Treatment program (EPSDT); lead poisoning; and environmental health. Environmental health programs include food and lodging sanitation, animal control, vector control, and general sanitation.[16]

Mental Health Agencies. Include a basic description of organizational structure, source of funding, and level of care provided.

Example 2–28a. The Crescent County Mental Health Department provides categorical programs in mental health for children and adults, mental retardation, and substance abuse. Each of the categorical programs offers outpatient, inpatient, day / night, emergency, and consultation and education services. Funds are derived from county, state, federal, and private sources.

Example 2–28b. Midland County Mental Health Center provides services in the broad categories of mental illness, mental retardation, substance abuse, vocational rehabilitation, and crises services. Inpatient care, prevention services, day treatment, and follow-up care are provided.

A state-supported psychiatric hospital as well as several private psychiatric hospitals are located within Midland County. Many changes have faced the Center in terms of services and funding. Costs of health care and federal block grants have greatly impacted on service provision. Community and governmental funds support the Mental Health Center. Many services are provided under contractual agreement with other agencies.

Voluntary Health Organizations. List the voluntary health organizations and describe their recent activities.

Example 2–29a. Crescent County is fortunate to have numerous voluntary health organizations based in and around Rapid City. Organizations such as the Cancer Society, Arthritis Center, Alcoholics Anonymous, Central Drug Council, Red Cross, Camp Longmont for Diabetics, Crises Action League, and Community Care are accessible to County residents. Most of these community service organizations have representation on the Crescent Community Council.

Although funding for the voluntary health organizations is obtained from the United Way, donations, membership dues, and private foundation funding, there has been considerable effort in avoiding duplication of services. There is an annual meeting of the Crescent Community Council during which community need as it compares to service availability is discussed. Task forces are sometimes developed to address an unmet need.

Recent projects have focused on daycare, community resources for emotionally disturbed children, chronic diseases, family counseling, and health promotion.

Example 2–29b. Metrocity and Midland County have numerous voluntary health organizations. Metrocity is noted for its history of providing services to low-income and isolated populations. Many municipalities have seen a growth in the number of voluntary agencies that are located outside Metrocity. Major voluntary health agencies (such as the American Heart Association, American Cancer Society, and the Lung Association) are located in Midland County. These agencies often have branch offices in the suburban communities.

Other Rural Health or Inner City Health Organizations. When information is available, describe other health organizations and their sources of funds.

Example 2–30a. Other than private physicians, the hospitals, and the health department, there are no other sources of primary health care in Crescent County. The northwest area of the county has been identified as a medically underserved area.

Example 2–30b. There are 10 community health centers in Midland County that are administered by the Metrocity Health Department. In addition, numerous health maintenance organizations have been developed in Midland County. The Midland County Hospital System provides medical care for the medically indigent population. These are the sources of primary health care in addition to the private medical care system.

Analysis of the Community's Social Assistance System

The next part of the community analysis is concerned with the social assistance system existing in the community. Descriptors of the social assistance system are found through investigation of the participation by the community in federal programs as well as programs developed locally.

Several questions concerning participation in *federal programs* must be answered. Does the community participate in major federal programs such as Medicare and Medicaid? Document programs in which the community does participate.

Example 2–31a. The social service programs in Crescent County are varied. They include Aid to Families with Dependent Children (AFDC), Medicaid, Food Stamps, and Medicare. All of these income maintenance programs, except Medicare, are administered by the county.

In addition to income maintenance programs, Crescent County provides the following social service programs: adoption, daycare for children, family planning, foster care for children and adults, health support, individual and family adjustment services, in-house services, protective services for children and adults, services for the blind, treatment services for alcoholics, delinquency prevention, services for the retarded and emotionally disturbed, counseling, and transportation. All of these programs are provided directly by Crescent County or upon contact with other appropriate agencies. In Crescent County, 1.77% of the population receive Aid to Families with Dependent Children, 3.99% receive Medicare, 3.30% receive Food Stamps, .03% receive Foster Care Services, 1.9% receive Information and Referral Services, and 1.57% receive Title XX Services. Crescent County ranks in the lower one third of counties in the State as far as the percent of county population receiving these services.

Example 2–31b. The percentage of residents of Midland County below the poverty level is 11.8%; 5.2% of the population is eligible for Medicaid. Per capita health care expenditures in Midland County are higher than the national level. The average monthly AFDC (Aid to Families with Dependent Children) payment per family is $289.00.

Locally generated programs are another descriptor of the social assistance system. Describe any *locally generated programs* that operate in the social assistance realm.

Example 2–32a. The primary, broad, community-based social assistance program in Crescent County is Community Care, Inc. Some of the services offered by this agency are housing information, employment counseling, crisis support (food, shelter, clothing, and fuel), referrals to appropriate medical services, and neighborhood development projects. Even though Community Care is a county-wide organization, the majority of the services are based in Rapid City.

Example 2–32b. Metrocity is noted for its locally generated social assistance programs. These programs are directed toward the inner city neighborhoods and specific social and health problems. The volunteer staff is from the neighborhoods and from the outside communities. Funding for these programs is usually from private and local contributions. The Urban Development Commission, Metrocity Church Council, Midland Neighborhood Councils Associations, and Metrocity Senior Citizens Advocacy Council are some of the largest, locally focused social assistance programs.

Community Diagnosis

Community diagnosis is the final part of the community analysis. Community diagnosis involves the synthesis of all information collected. It is designed to identify gaps between health status and the provision of health services within an area.

Community diagnosis includes four basic steps: (1) determining the state of health of the community, (2) determining the pattern of health service delivery in the community, (3) determining the relationship between health status and health care in the community, and (4) identifying and establishing the determinants of the major problems relating to health needs and resources in the community. During these four steps of diagnosis, the data collected in the community analysis are pulled together and major trends or problems are identified. At this point, populations that may share the trends or problems are determined. With the identification of major trends or problems and the populations that experience them, our understanding of the community is more than simply a list of facts and figures.

The community diagnosis identifies the segments of the population, the target populations, where health problems seem to be concentrated, and the related health problems of the target populations. The phrase "target population" refers to that portion of a community that is identified as a focus for a health education program. In other words, the target population consists of those individuals for whom the program(s) under consideration are designed and implemented. The definition of the target population enables individuals engaged in program planning and service delivery to distinguish intended program participants from those not targeted. Identification of a target population brings to light a group or groups of people with common needs and often common characteristics, so that programs are most cost effective and have greater potential to demonstrate measurable change after implementation.

In identifying the target population for health education, it is important to understand the perspective of the individuals involved in the planning process. What appears as a social problem to one group may not be perceived as such by another.[17] Health educators need to be particularly vigilant to ensure that their definitions of target groups reflect careful analysis of the group's problems through the eyes *of that group.*[18] It is easy to misdiagnose community health problems by failing to understand the perspective of community members. A proper "diagnosis" of a community and subsequent target groups is ensured by involving target group members in the information gathering and diagnostic phases of program planning.

Determining the Community's State of Health

In determining the state of health of the community, the data collected in the community analysis must be interpreted. Raw data must be transformed into rates to begin to understand how the community compares to other similar communities or to the state as a whole. The data are not helpful unless they provide a basis for comparison.

While developing a community diagnosis, we may work with several types of data. Some data may have been gathered by using tightly controlled techniques such as sample surveys. These data, sometimes referred to as "hard" data, are more reliable; that is, if we use the same data-gathering instrument in a different community, the same type of responses may be expected. This type of data gathering allows planners to compare communities. On the other hand, more informal data-gathering techniques may have been used, such as direct observation, open-ended interviews, or the key informant approach in which the results may be biased by the observer or the respondent. Informal data-gathering techniques produce "soft" data that are not replicable, yet provide valuable insight into the community and the opinions of its residents. All available data should be considered in pulling together a statement or diagnosis on the community's state of health.

The community analysis was a data-gathering process that permitted the collection of vital statistics such as live birth rate, fetal mortality rate, infant mortality rate, neonatal death rate, and overall death rate. We then investigated the death rates further to see if the cause was infectious diseases or chronic diseases. We considered the causes of death and the morbidity related to certain diseases, including occupational diseases. In the community diagnosis, we build upon the health status data gathered during the community analysis and draw specific conclusions about the health of the population in the area. For example, we may conclude that the community has a high rate of infant mortality, chronic diseases, or infectious diseases by comparing the community's rates for particular factors to rates for similar communities or for a larger unit such as the county or state of which the community under study is a part.

Example 2–33a. Vital statistics indicate that Crescent County fares better than the state as a whole in the number of deaths of children under 1 year of age. However, death rates attributable to particular chronic diseases are higher for Crescent County than for the state. Specifically, deaths due to infective and parasitic diseases, neoplasia, diseases of the circulatory and endocrine systems, and nutritional and metabolic diseases occur at a higher rate than for the state.

Example 2–33b. Midland County is a growing and prosperous area. Certain segments of the population experience more health problems than the general population. Death rates caused by most chronic diseases and homicide are particularly high when compared with national death rates. Perinatal and infant death rates are also high.

Determining the Pattern of Health Services

By determining the pattern of health services in the community, we can assess the resources that provide health and medical care. As the community analysis indicated, basic health services are offered in most urban communities or counties. These include hospitals, private physicians, a health department, and voluntary health organizations. In addition, the number of medical, allied-health, and public health professionals as compared to the total population is considered a measure of available services. Not only should we consider the availability of facilities and health providers but also their accessibility. Accessibility is a measure of the extent to which community residents can obtain the available services. For example, community health services may not be accessible because of geographic distance, hours of operation, qualifying criteria, or backlog of appointments. Areas of the community may be considered medically underserved on the basis of either availability of services or manpower. From a study of the health services within a community, we should be able to determine whether the entire population has access to health services. We may find that particular age, racial, or ethnic groups or people living in a particular area may be isolated from health care.

It should be easy to gather data on the available health services within the community; however, these data should not be accepted without question. As with health status data, many issues related to health services can be discovered only after talking directly with providers, the staff as well as management, and community residents.

The process of discovering the intricacies of the health services within a community, such as why a facility was built where it was, or who actually decides what services to offer, is a continuing one. Knowledge and understanding of the community will certainly increase as the analysis process continues.

Example 2–34a. In Crescent County, there are two hospitals, a health department, numerous voluntary health organizations, a mental health department, nursing homes, and a variety of medical and health personnel. Closer study shows that the majority of these services are located within Rapid City. The residents of Bryson's Fork are considered medically underserved. Even though there is a variety of medical and health personnel within the county, the physician-to-population ratio is 1 to 828 as compared to 1 to 789 for the State. In terms of health education within Crescent County, minimal health education coverage within the health department is minimal. There are also no comprehensive health education programs within the hospitals or schools, even though interest in health education has been expressed in each of these settings.

Example 2–34b. The health care services available in Midland County appear adequate. Metrocity has HMOs and primary care centers, the hospital, the health department, and private providers that offer health care services to residents. Several inner city neighborhoods do not have ready access to these services.

Investigating the Relationship between Health Status and Health Care

In the third step of the community diagnosis, we investigate the relationship between health status and health care in the community. Health indicators for potential target populations are correlated. Populations with health status problems are compared to the populations for whom services are not available or accessible. We may find a direct correlation between the two; if so, this probably indicates a population in greatest need. This population may or may not be the population for which a health education program is indicated. It is possible that an educational program directed toward the population in greatest need may not promote any desirable change within that particular population. Sometimes the population in greatest need will not have the resources to change immediately. Designing an initial health education program for a population in severe need may lead the program toward failure and the population into distress. More study is required to assess this possibility. Although health education programs can be planned and successfully implemented for populations with varying intensities of need, thorough analysis of the population and its resources will indicate which programs are suited for that population.

Care must be taken in assuming a direct relationship between health services and health status. We must consider whether the lack of particular services or the provision of those services will make an impact on the health status of the population. We may discover, for example, that proper diet or increased exercise may affect particular health indices more than the provision of medical services. In contrast, we may find that the provision of emergency medical transport vehicles may decrease the death rates attributable to motor vehicle accidents. Unfortunately, many health programs are evaluated on the basis of the numbers of services delivered, such as hypertension screenings or number of educational sessions presented, rather than on the actual health outcome.

Target group identification is the most important outcome of comparing health status to health services. If we determine that a particular group has a particular problem, we may find either that there is no service to address that problem, that there is a service but the target population does not use it, that there is no service available but the target population seeks services elsewhere, or that there is a service and the population uses it. Indications of the health education program(s) needed to alleviate the health problem now become clear. For example, if there is no service to address a need, we may design an educational program directed at helping the population, our target population for the program, express their need to community decision-makers or health providers so that plans can be made for providing that service. If there is a service but the target population does not use it, we may consider designing a health education program that includes strategies for increasing attendance. Many possibilities for programs exist, but so far data are not sufficiently available to determine exactly how or why the program should be designed. We still lack adequate information for planning the specifics of our health education program. We still have only speculations concerning a target population and program.

Example 2–35a. In Crescent County, the major health status problems identified through the community analysis included higher death rates per 100,000 than for the entire state resulting from: (1) infective and parasitic diseases; (2) neoplasia; (3) endocrine, nutritional, and metabolic diseases; and (4) diseases of the circulatory system. Crescent County also had higher rates per 100,000 for encephalitis, Rocky Mountain spotted fever, and rubella. Finally, large numbers of individuals employed in manufacturing industries sustained occupational injuries.

From the community analysis, we can speculate that limited health resources and a high physician-to-population ratio are factors related to the overall death rate per 100,000 population, which is higher than for the state as a whole. Limited health resources may also be related to the high mortality and morbidity rates attributable to particular diseases. We can also speculate that mortality and morbidity rates reflect the lack of health education programs in the community as well as health care agencies, because all of the listed health problems have individual behavioral components.

Our data are not sufficient to determine which part(s) of the county, or in other words, what specific community, experiences the problems most severely. If we could plot, for example, the communities where individuals lived who experienced particular problems, then we would perhaps have sufficient data to warrant particular services or programs based in one community.

Example 2–35b. The health care services available to most Midland County residents are adequate, and yet the rates for most leading causes of death are higher than those for the entire state. The quantity of health services bears no direct relationship to health status.

Identifying Major Community Health Issues

The fourth step of the community diagnosis involves identifying and establishing the determinants of the major issues and problems related to health needs and resources of the community. During this step, we identify factors related to health resources and needs within the community. Such factors may include the background of the community and its economic, political, and social structure. In addition, we may utilize data on geographic or climate characteristics to determine why the community has particular problems. For example, high death rates attributable to hypothermia may be related to low socio-economic levels, high numbers of elderly individuals, and an extremely cold climate. We may also want to consider what community services or resources are available to confront the problem as we investigate determinants of the major problems.

As the process of community diagnosis becomes more and more complicated, knowledge of the target population should become more detailed. At this point in community diagnosis, we should have an idea of potential target population(s), the related needs, and the available resources, and we should have started assessing the determinants of the problems related to all three factors. Even though we will certainly have generated more questions than answers in this step of community diagnosis, we should begin to have ideas of health education programs needed by particular populations and where the program should be implemented within the community. After we have identified possible target populations, we may need to inquire into specific characteristics of the proposed target populations for the planning of health education programs. These characteristics or determinants may include such factors as education, age, race, sex, geographic location, behavioral attributes, or religious beliefs. We could probably begin our process of analysis again with our target population; however, involvement with the target population or community need only be to the extent necessary for assuring that the program planned on the basis of previously gathered data is as solid as possible.

Example 2–36a. In addition to obvious health status problems and maldistribution of services, · we can determine other factors from the community analysis that would impact on the health status of Crescent County. The general socioeconomic status of Crescent County is better than average for the state. Fewer individuals and families receive social assistance than in most counties. Transition from farm to factory employment is steady; the number of women entering the work force has increased; the major source of employment is manufacturing industries; and overall, the county is growing in terms of both total population and the number of industries being established. Although these factors account for an increase in socioeconomic status, their impact on health status is not clear. An increase in the socioeconomic status may also account for an increase in death rates attributable to neoplasia and disease of the circulatory system as well as the high numbers of occupational injuries.

The low educational level among county residents, the lack of comprehensive health education programs, the lack of public transportation systems, the high number of residents who work, and the high number who work outside the county may also affect the health status of the population. These factors may be determinants of the high death rates attributable to infective and parasitic diseases as well as the high number of cases of encephalitis, Rocky Mountain spotted fever, and rubella.

As with trying to determine the relationship between health status and health services, specifying the determinants of the major health problems within Crescent County is difficult and speculative at this point. More study is needed to identify specific determinants of health status for the target populations.

Several potential target populations are indicated from our community analysis. A potential target group may include (1) the community of Bryson's Fork and other communities located in the northwest part of the county who are isolated from health services. We do not know yet if particular health problems are higher in this area than in other areas of the county. Other potential target populations may be (2) health department patrons, especially home health care recipients, individuals who should be immunized for rubella and those at risk of chronic diseases such as hypertension, cancer, diabetes, and glaucoma; (3) health department personnel who are responsible for home health, chronic disease, and health education programs; (4) employees of manufacturing industries who are at risk of occupational injuries; and (5) residents of a geographic area within the city just south of the interstate who utilize the emergency rooms of the hospitals as a primary source of medical care. There may be other target populations for health education programs within Crescent County that have not yet been identified.

Example 2–36b. The accessibility of health care services and the socio-economic and environmental conditions for residents of Midland County are potential areas of future study. Targeting of programs would include: (1) isolated neighborhoods; (2) residents at risk of developing or who already have chronic diseases; (3) major work groups, especially those related to manufacturing industries; and (4) pregnant women and young children.

COLLECTING DATA FROM THE COMMUNITY

The community diagnosis is only as adequate as the data on which it is based. The health educator must decide what and how data will be gathered. Some information can be obtained from assorted public documents such as the U.S. Census as well as from state and local vital statistics or demographic reports. Other information may require the input of other professionals skilled in data collection in such subjects as designing the data collection instruments, the procedures for analyzing the data, and the plan for presenting the findings. The health educator must determine whether such assistance is needed to perform an adequate community analysis.

Certain data can only be obtained by questioning members of the community. Several techniques may be used for gaining additional insight into the interactions among community members. The techniques subsequently outlined are, in order of increasing complexity, and include cost considerations.

Key Informant Approach

Sometimes referred to as the "grapevine" approach, the key informant approach involves the use of information collected from knowledgeable individuals, "key informants," to provide additional insight into problems of a specific group.[17] The concept underlying this technique is that certain individuals in a group, by virtue of their experience, profession, or elected office, can contribute valuable information about issues involving a community. This information may help us to understand a problem more fully by presenting a different perception of it.

The key informant approach involves simple and relatively inexpensive procedures. The information that is collected can represent a wide variety of perspectives on a single issue, and the key informants themselves may become valuable assets to the program planning and implementation process in the future. The steps to be followed in using this approach follow.

1. Identify the characteristics of key informants who would likely have insight into the issues under study.
2. Select potential key informants and make an initial contact to determine whether they desire to participate.
3. Determine the specific information you want to obtain and the specific questions you plan to ask the key informants. The questions may be structured into a questionnaire or interview. After constructing the instrument (questionnaire or interview), pretest it by conducting a pilot test.
4. Administer the instrument, person-to-person (interview), by mail, or over the telephone. Depending on the nature of the issue, the community, and characteristics of the key informants themselves, one of these methods may prove superior. In some cases, a combination of the methods may be used.
5. Tabulate the data collected and draw any possible conclusions. Any conclusions drawn must be supported by the data collected. A more rigorous survey must be designed and implemented to provide data that will enable inferences to be drawn.

Because the key informant approach encompasses the collection of data from individuals presumed to represent different perspectives on the nature of an issue relative to a specific target group, remember that the informants do not have *all* the information pertaining to the issue, but only respond from their own point of view. In addition, the key informants chosen from the community do not necessarily represent *all* important informants. The informants selected are those who agreed to cooperate; thus, the selection process is biased. Consequently, information collected through use of the key informant process should be evaluated carefully.

Community Forum Approach

Another method of collecting information is to conduct a community forum through which relevant issues may be discussed. In this forum, the discussion may be guided in an attempt to understand better the subtle processes influencing a problem under study. The forum approach also allows for interchange among various community forces, and has the potential of facilitating meaningful communication among individuals of different convictions. Some community problems may actually be solved through use of a community forum.

From the point of view of the health educator, the community forum is very economical. Health educators can also understand the interrelationships among various forces in the community. Its major limitation is that those present at a forum, much less those speaking, rarely represent a target group or community. It is difficult to persuade a truly representative cross-section of the area to attend a community forum because their interests tend to vary greatly. Depending on the community in question as well as the issue for discussion, religious groups, labor organizations, civic organizations, or other community organizations such as a PTA may prove helpful in organizing a well-attended community forum.

Focus Group Approach

The focus group approach is a marketing technique used to understand the behavior of consumers.[19] These groups are used to identify attitudes and other psychologic issues related to the product under study. Focus groups are often used to gain initial data to help guide the design of more intense research. This technique may be particularly helpful in a needs assessment process.

A focus group usually comprises 6 to 12 individuals of similar cultural backgrounds. The moderator directs the session and asks questions to solicit group reactions to the issue of concern. Usually only one major area is addressed by a single focus group.

The moderator develops and directs the group. Participation by all group members is encouraged. The session usually lasts about two hours and is usually taped or video-taped. Later analysis allows interpretation of the opinions and behaviors of the focus group participants. Because the members of the focus group were selected on the basis of their characteristics similar to a broader group, generalizations are often drawn about the larger population's attitudes or practices. This applicability to a general population can be helpful to health educators when developing or testing new programs.

Sample Survey Approach

Properly done, a sample survey is the most comprehensive way to develop a valid perception of the health needs of a community. These surveys can be tailor-made to fit varying populations and their subpopulations. Estimates of error can be selected, and the survey procedures can be modified to produce results with a predetermined level of accuracy. Unfortunately, high quality sample surveys are an expensive approach to assessing the needs of a community.

Because many health educators are not sufficiently trained to design and implement detailed sample surveys, expert statistical consultation should be obtained. We cannot overemphasize the importance of acquiring expert consultation in the area of sample surveying. The design of surveys requires an understanding of the basic nature of the inquiry beginning with the initial planning of the survey instrument. Conducting a survey requires more than devising a survey instrument, selecting the group(s) of people for administration, and collecting the data. To produce defensible results from a sample survey, plan carefully—with the help of an expert.

To engage a consultant in the area of sample surveys, prepare some basic information. First, what population is considered a "universe" population? The population from which you select your respondents is the population that you want your survey to describe. Second, is the desired information best collected by using a self-administered questionnaire or by an interviewer? Third, and perhaps most importantly how much money is available? The interviewers usually need to be paid; there will probably be charges for duplicating the survey instruments; you may need funds for analyzing the data once they are collected; and finally, you probably will have to pay the consultant. Given these queries and expenses, you might decide to use another method to assess needs. Remember, when considering sample surveys, anything not worth doing well is really not worth doing at all!

On the basis of further study of available resources, verification of need, and assessment of target population behaviors, we may design our health education programs to address the needs of one or more target populations. The likelihood of program implementation, the educational readiness of target populations, and many other factors may have a direct influence on the outcome of the program planning process. Through identifying a target population and the related needs, resources, and determinants of the problems, we have laid the foundation for a health education program plan. Certainly many questions resulting from the community diagnosis are unanswered, so our next steps are imperative. We must verify our diagnosis with the target population if they are not intensely involved in the process of analysis and diagnosis. After that, we can ask additional questions related to the target population and then plan the specifics of our program.

REFERENCES

1. Green, L.W.: Evaluation and measurement: some dilemmas for health education. Am. J. Public Health, *67*(2):155, 1977.
2. Blum, H.L.: Planning for Health: Development and Application of Social Change Theory. New York, Human Sciences Press, 1974.
3. Jones, W.R.: Finding Community: A Guide to Community Research and Action. Palo Alto, California, James E. Freel, 1971.
4. Cassel, J.C.: Community Diagnosis. *In* Community Medicine in Developing Countries. Edited by A.R. Omran. New York, Springer Publishing, 1974.
5. Agger, R.E., Goldrich, D., and Swanson, B.: The Rulers and the Ruled: Power and Impotence in American Communities. New York, Wiley, 1964.
6. Webber, M.M. (ed.): The urban place and the non-place urban realm. *In* Explorations into Urban Structures. Philadelphia, University of Pennsylvania, 1964.
7. Hochstrasser, D.L., Trapp, J.W., and Dockal, N.: Community Health Study Outline. Lexington, Kentucky, Unpublished manuscript, Department of Community Medicine, College of Medicine, Medical Center University of Kentucky, June, 1968.
8. Warren, R.B., and Warren, D.I.: The Neighborhood Organizer's Handbook. Notre Dame, Indiana, University of Notre Dame Press, 1977.
9. Nelson, R.E. (ed.): Illinois—Land and Life in the Prairie State. Dubuque, Iowa, Kendall / Hunt, 1978.
10. U.S. Bureau of the Census: Statistical Abstract of the United States, 1986. 106th Ed. Washington, D.C. 1985.
11. Shryock, H.S., and Siegel, J.S.: The Methods and Materials of Demography, Vol. 1. Washington, D.C., U.S. Department of Commerce, Social and Economic Statistics Administration, Bureau of the Census, May, 1973.
12. Miller, C.A., and Moos, M.: local Health Departments—Fifteen Case Studies. Washington, D.C., American Public Health Association, 1981.
13. American Heart Association: 1986 Heart Facts. Dallas, 1985.
14. State of North Carolina, Department of Human Resources, Division of Health Services: Memorandum to Local Health Directors from W.B. Jones, M.D. regarding chronic disease program planning workshops. Raleigh, January 27, 1978.
15. USDHEW, PHS, CDC, NIOSH: Occupational Diseases: A Guide to Their Recognition. USDHP Pub. No. 77-181, 1977.
16. North Carolina Vital Statistics, Vol. I: Raleigh, 1977.
17. Rossi, P.H., Freeman, H.E., and Wright, S.R.: Evaluation: A Systematic Approach. Beverly Hills, Sage, 1979.
18. Paul, B.D. (ed.): Health, Culture and Community. New York, Russell Sage, 1955.
19. Folch-Lyon, E., and Trost, J.F.: Conducting focus group sessions. *In* Studies in Family Planning. Vol. 12. No. 12. New York, Population Council, 1981.

3

Focusing Program Development

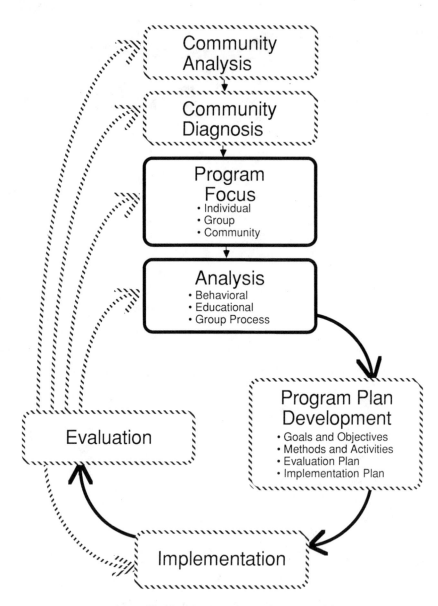

The Health Education / Promotion Planning Model.

3

Focusing Program
Development

Through community analysis and diagnosis, health planners may identify target populations, their health problems and other issues related to health in the community. The diagnosis may be accurate and provide an appropriate assessment of the needs of the population. Program plans may seem to flow naturally from the diagnosis. In most instances, however, the community analysis provides global descriptions of the health problems amenable to health education. The analytic process is rarely precise enough to allow planning for health education and promotion without additional study of the target population.

EXTENDING COMMUNITY ANALYSIS

The community analysis may conclude without having a specific health education focus identified for the target population. In other words, the conclusions reached in a community analysis are broad and can be used by a variety of planners, i.e., facility planners, community development specialists, or agency administrators. Those individuals seeking to plan health education and health promotion programs need to use these conclusions as a starting point for a more detailed investigation of health-related knowledge, attitudes, and behaviors. This detailed investigation is intended to focus the planning process.

By taking a series of steps, a health planner can extend the planning process beyond a general community health focus to a specific health education and promotion focus. These steps include (1) determining whether the group or organization contemplating planning has the resources necessary to complete the job; (2) verifying the health problems and issues with the target population; (3) establishing program goals; (4) defining the specific target group behaviors that the program will seek to influence; and (5) identifying the appropriate focus for the educational and promotional activities of the program (individual, group, or community-wide).

Resources for Planning

The conclusions generated from the community analysis may or may not be sufficiently interesting or appropriate to merit the attention of a group or organization that can undertake program planning. Considering whether to proceed with planning involves deciding whether the health problems of the target population are relevant to the skills and interests of the planners. In other words, the program planners and the target group must, to some extent, have mutual goals. For example, individuals whose goals include the promotion of occupational health might be best suited to planning programs aimed at reducing back injuries in a given work force.

Those persons considering program planning must also consider their own resources in relation to the planning. The resources may be in the form of sufficient time, staffing, educational materials, or funding. (The specific resources needed to put health education and promotion programs into effect are discussed in depth in Chapter 5.)

Verifying Issues with the Target Group

One of the basic questions resulting from a community analysis is whether the analytic process explored the problems and concerns held by community members. Despite considerable efforts, the community analysis may have been so narrowly focused that the concerns of many community residents were not examined. It is necessary to verify conclusions derived through community analysis with the members of the target populations. It is more likely that the target population will actively participate in a program designed to address a community problem if they see themselves as having that problem. Additionally, if community residents believe that a problem is of sufficient gravity to merit their concern, they are more likely to support efforts to correct it.

Concerns of health care providers, including health educators, and community leaders are often significant in planning for health care services. A common assumption is that professionals in the health fields know what is best for the community's health care. Such a perception may give rise to just criticism of health programs because the opinions of the providers of health care concerned with community needs do not automatically represent the needs of the community. The needs of the entire community often conflict with the needs of specific target groups.

Community analysis may also fail to explore adequately the concerns of community members if it minimizes or ignores the needs of those who provide services. Occasionally, community analysis is limited to information collected from community residents (consumers). Data from these consumers must be balanced, however, with input from health providers. Providers commonly have information about community health problems that is helpful to consumers in resolving problems. Providers may also participate in resolution of community health problems. Finally, providers usually have their own needs and resources that must be acknowledged when addressing a health problem within the community. The needs of providers and consumers must be included if an accurate picture of community health problems is to be developed.

The community analysis format directs data collection from many different points of view. Unless specific attention is directed toward health concerns, the data provided by the community analysis may lead to a wide variety of conclusions that are unrelated to health concerns. Lack of focus is perhaps the most salient criticism of the community analysis approach in program planning. The community analysis process considers such a wide variety of concerns that specific issues may become lost in a sea of statistics.

Good indicators of community needs are "felt needs" of target populations.[1, 2] Felt needs are those areas of concern most often articulated by the target population.[3, 4] Felt needs are the most pressing problems experienced by groups and individuals in the target population, and they usually reflect the problems of immediate concern. The felt needs of the target population, however, do not necessarily represent the concerns of the entire community. Results of community analysis, when based on thorough exploration of issues, may help to place felt needs in perspective. In this way, these results are useful as an educational tool. Health educators may use the results of a community analysis in educating the target group about where their health problems originate. The process may help to improve cohesiveness in the community. Members of the target population need to understand that problems are rarely faced by only one person, or one group of people, and that solutions to problems are often complex.

When seeking input to verify the results of community analysis, independent sources of information should be included, that is, sources of information not used in the original community analysis. If independent sources agree on community health problems, then by virtue of the agreement the educator may feel more confident about the conclusions of the community analysis. If opinions from certain community leaders were used to generate information to be used in the community analysis, opinions from different community leaders should be sought out for verification. An independent source of information either confirms or refutes the original source, allowing conclusions to be tested. Suppose the key informant approach was used as part of the community analysis in Chapter 2. To verify the conclusions of the community analysis, *different* key informants would be identified.[4] If these new informants agreed with the conclusions, and thereby implicitly agreed with the original key informants, then a source of verification was obtained. On the other hand, if new key informants disagreed with the conclusions of the community analysis, the planner would have to determine whether the disagreement meant that the conclusions were wrong or that key informants have different perceptions. In either case, a stronger base of understanding is built of how the community and target population function.

Where statistical information from official sources was used in the community analysis, verification presents a different problem. Official statistics are commonly accepted at face value. Community analyses may also be limited by the age of the data on which conclusions were based. Depending on the nature of the information, public health data may be grossly inaccurate by the time they are published. This problem is particularly troublesome in communities experiencing rapid growth. The influx of new people into rapid growth areas often makes public health statistics questionable. If the data on which the community analysis was based have changed between the time when the original conclusions were drawn and the present, then naturally the conclusions may be misleading.

Independent sources of information that can be used to verify official statistics are difficult to identify. One approach, however, is to identify trends within the official statistics and seek out other data that might confirm or question the existence of the trend. For example, an increasing or decreasing birth rate in a community might also be reflected in adoption service statistics, activity of private medical practitioners and public family planning agencies in providing contraception and abortion services, and the percentage of women between the ages of 15 and 44 years in the population.

By verifying the problems within the community, predetermined by the community analysis, an accurate perception of community health problems is sought. The areas of concern of the target population must be explored sufficiently to understand the dynamics of the health problems that exist. If the analysis of the community is not verified, then programs may be produced that do not meet the needs of the community.

ESTABLISHING PROGRAM GOALS

If the community analysis is validated, the next step in program planning is to develop a set of program goal statements. Program goal statements correspond to the problems delineated by the community analysis and are usually indexed to specific target groups. These statements represent the first concrete step toward planning programs for specific community health problems. In program planning for community health education, two sets of goal statements, program goals and educational goals are eventually developed. *Program goals* are directed toward a particular community health problem, and are designed to outline the expected achievements of the program. *Educational goals* are statements that describe resolution of health problems through educational strategies. Education is usually only a component of health programs. For this reason, educational goals are commonly dictated by program goals (see Fig. 3–1).

Goals are statements that reflect what programs are intended to produce.[5] They are the "intended consequences of a program."[6] In developing statements to describe goals, issues are clarified and flexible guidelines for planning are established. Because of the need for flexibility at this stage in planning, goal statements tend to be descriptive, global statements of what is intended. Goal statements also direct further inquiry into the planning

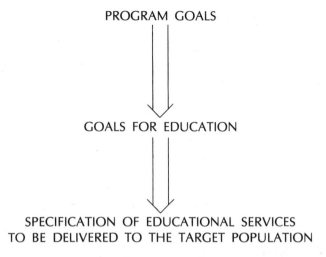

Fig. 3-1. The relationship between program goals, educational goals and meeting the needs of the target population.

process. The orientation is toward "improving health status" in the community, through planning and implementing programs for remediation of specific community health concerns in particular segments of the population.

In the analyses of Crescent County and Midland County (see Chapter 2), we identified some potential target populations: Bryson's Fork and the surrounding hamlets, isolated urban neighborhoods, health department patrons (particularly home health care recipients), health department personnel, employees in manufacturing industries, individuals with chronic disease, and persons who use the emergency room at local hospitals as a source of primary care. Tentative program goal statements for each of these target populations can be developed.

1. Bryson's Fork and surrounding hamlets will have increased access to health care services.
2. Urban neighborhoods will have accessible, available health care.
3. Users of home health care services provided through the Crescent County Health Department will have a defined health education component in the care they receive.
4. The staff of the Crescent County Health Department will include planned health education in their duties where appropriate.
5. Crescent County residents at high risk for accidental injury due to their occupation will have a reduced rate of accidental injury.
6. Individuals at risk for chronic disease will participate in a health promotion program.
7. Families and individuals who use the emergency rooms in Crescent County hospitals for non-emergency health care will use private physicians as their source of health care.

Each program will also have educational goals; with changes in knowledge, attitudes, or behaviors as their focus. These statements will be developed in the process of planning the specific health education activities to be applied in each situation.

DEFINING TARGET GROUP BEHAVIOR

Failing to specify adequately the behavior or behaviors that need to be changed is one of the most fundamental errors made in planning community health education and promotion programs. The focus of programs in health education and promotion is on behavioral change. The specific nature of the health problem and the target population(s) must be clearly understood initially and then described completely through community diagnosis. The target populations then verify these problems, which ensures that the community health problems identified through community analysis are indeed those perceived as important by the target population.[7, 8]

Merely identifying and verifying a community health problem or issue is insufficient for continuing the process of program planning in health education and promotion. Additional issues are those of identifying who experiences the problem, the behaviors of those individuals or groups, the mechanisms that maintain the behavior(s), and determining whether the desired change has taken place. The circumstances under which the health problem occurs must also be carefully delineated. Behaviors are usually the targets for change through health education and promotion programs, but are only a part of the development of health problems.

The identified health problem may not be a result of the actions or inactions of the target population. The problem may be a result of the actions or inactions of health providers, politicians, or others. Health professionals tend to see clients or patients as persons in need of services without looking critically at the type and quality of service provided. In many cases, clients' problems are really their problems in dealing with their community's health care delivery system. For example, the Crescent County residents who use the emergency room for routine health care may do so because it is more convenient. They may also use the emergency room in an effort to gain access to regular medical care from practitioners who are not accepting new patients.

Describing specific behaviors involved with community health problems requires a detailed explanation of the actions or inactions of the clients and / or health providers associated with the problem identified. The behavior or behaviors may be very simple and involve one individual in a clear-cut situation. More commonly, the behaviors involve the individual, the family, the community, and the health provider(s) intertwined in a complex relationship. In the latter situation, isolating the specific behavior or behaviors of interest may be difficult. For example, residents of Crescent County who are employed in manufacturing industries are at higher risk of industrial accidents than any other group in the county. Defining the specific behaviors related to industrial accidents in this setting would involve the accident victim, the management of the plant where the accident occurred, and the other workers in the plant. The network of factors related to chronic disease in Midland County is highly variable, depending on the individual and his or her environment. Unraveling behaviors of all these parties to identify the specific behavioral mechanisms included in a health problem could be very complicated. To specify the behaviors, data are systematically collected from those involved with the accident.

Health educators traditionally have considered the health education process as a mixture of knowledge, attitudes, and behaviors.[1] The problem under scrutiny may be based in a lack of knowledge, an uncompromising attitude, or unrewarding behavior patterns. In most instances, health problems dealt with by health educators include all three components. It is highly unlikely that a single underlying relationship will be uncovered. Many behavioral patterns that result in positive health consequences over the long term are difficult to maintain over the short term. A diet that contains excessive calories is likely to be satisfying in the short term because it tastes good and reduces feelings of hunger that are uncomfortable, but will result in added body weight if continued over the long term. A restrictive diet may be unrewarding in the short term, but will lead to a satisfying long-term outcome.

It is tempting to hold the conviction that people are rational, and that destructive health behaviors are the result of gaps in knowledge. If this were true, however, then health education programs would be successful simply by producing information for clients in such a way that the gaps in knowledge were filled. Unfortunately, most people are not rational all the time; rather, they are *rationalizing* all the time.[9] They are not motivated always to be correct in the things that they do; rather, they are motivated to *believe* that they are correct. Because of this quirk of human nature, relying on information alone in health education programs usually leaves us far short of our goals.

If knowledge does not produce good explanations for the behaviors seen in community health problems, then attitudes should be considered. Attitudes supply valuable information for program planning. For example, the target population may place great trust and value in indigenous "home remedies." Potential problems are avoided by including these perceptions in decisions about the content of the program. Indigenous attitudes should be incorporated into the program wherever possible, or potential reactions in the target population are likely to occur.

Attitudes are really a form of nonverbal behavior. They do not necessarily match with motor behavior. In some cases behaviors reflect the attitudes of groups or individuals. Most often, however, attitudes are like a piece of a puzzle. They may help to explain parts of the observed behaviors but do not provide suffcient insight to be used in planning without other data.

The desired change sets the stage for writing objectives for the problem plan. In deciding on the desired change(s), consideration of the amount of change possible within a given time frame, and the resources necessary to achieve the change is essential. Making sound judgments about making change necessitates a close look at the behaviors of the target population and the providers.

When data have been collected and analyzed and the problem under consideration is better understood a target behavior or outcome can be identified.[10] The target behavior or outcome should be one that provides good "economy" for the proposed community health education program, which means identifying one that provides the best chance of a good outcome from the program over a reasonable period of time. It is tempting to select the most irritating or the most obvious outcome or behavior, but in fact it may be a false economy, like being "penny wise and dollar foolish."[11] Some criteria for the selection of behaviors or outcomes may emerge from the answers to the following questions:[12]

1. Will dealing with this behavior / outcome provide the best chance for attaining long-term change? Is the behavior an early link in a chain that will ultimately lead to the long-term change desired?
2. Will dealing with this behavior / outcome involve curtailing a positive aspect of the client's life?
3. Is this behavior / outcome so pervasive in our society that avoidance would be next to impossible for anyone?
4. Will dealing with this behavior / outcome increase the skills of the client?
5. Is this behavior / outcome one that can be dealt with on a contractual basis between the health educator and the client?

It is apparent that the behavior / outcome should be one that seeks to influence behaviors or outcomes over the long term, and not merely a "band-aid" approach. The behavior / outcome selected should be one for which changes can be measured easily in positive terms. The initial behavior / outcome selected should not be so complex or such an integral part of life that a change will represent a cause for despair in the client. Finally, the behavior / outcome should be one that is amenable to arranging a contractual agreement between the health educator and the client(s).

When we make a decision about events or outcomes to use in program planning, the stage is set for writing specific behavioral objectives. Selection of a target behavior or outcome commits us to developing a program to change a specific aspect of the behaviors of our clients. If we select a particular outcome, the health education program will be designed to avoid development of the outcome and will focus on behavior. Ideally we would select events (behaviors) that would prevent the development of an undesirable outcome. In most cases, however, the variables that are associated with prevention are the most difficult to use for program planning. In addition, prevention of an outcome may not be the desire of the target population. The target population may be more concerned with attacking the outcome directly and may be convinced that the outcome cannot be prevented, or, more commonly, that the cost of prevention is too high. This phenomenon is common when dealing with clients who have chronic diseases. For example, in developing a program to prevent early death from heart disease, we may use several variables to analyze our target population—a group of men, aged 45 to 50 years, with hypertension—and derive a host of behavior chains that deal with behaviors such as weight control, smoking, and psychic stress. If we focus on weight control as an outcome, we could use a self-report measure—a 24-hour dietary recall—to collect preliminary data on eating behavior. On the basis of the results of our observations and the self-report measures, we might decide that our group should gradually increase the time and intensity of exercise and begin a calorie-based program of weight reduction. On this plan, our target population should lose 1 to 2 pounds per week. When presented with the plan, the target population might likely reject the program. The amount of time and effort required to exercise regularly and the added stress from concern over caloric intake may seem too much to pay for a greater chance of a long life. The cost of prevention in this situation is simply too great for the target population. To make programs such as this succeed, positive short-term consequences must be made available to the participants.[13]

MODELS FOR BEHAVIORAL ASSESSMENT

Health educators are committed to the notion that health education should result in desirable behavior change. The first step in changing behavior is assessing the behavior or behaviors that need to be changed, and the social context in which they occur. Only after the specific behavior(s) that need changing have been assessed can methods to accomplish the change be selected or devised. Psychologists, psychiatrists, and many others concerned with the study of behavior itself have expended tremendous effort toward defining behavior. To know whether a person's behavior is out of the range of "normal" behavior, mental health professionals realize that they need more than their own judgment. Consequently, voluminous literature is available explaining how behavior is assessed and characterized.[14–17] For our purposes in planning programs for community health education, it is useful to consider health "behavior" as either *events* or *outcomes*.[18] An event is a behavior. An outcome is the result of behavior or behaviors.

When looking at behavior in health education, rarely is one single event or one single behavior involved. Health problems, as in the cases of most other human problems, seldom occur independently. That is, when a behavior occurs (an event), it is usually related in some way to something that already occurred or is to follow. Another way of expressing this idea is to consider behaviors in chains, and not as events that are unrelated to other events or outcomes. In medical settings, most patients, especially those with chronic conditions, represent outcomes of chains of events. Regardless of whether the focus is on the health concerns of an individual, a group, or an entire system for the delivery of health care, the consideration of events or outcomes provides valuable data that can be used for program planning. Some examples follow.

1. When Mr. Adams is examined in the outpatient clinic, he is at least 20% overweight. Is his weight an event or an outcome? Mr. Adams'

weight is an outcome of a chain of behaviors that includes eating excess calories for the amount of energy required for his body. The events would be the behaviors that make up the chain.

2. Mrs. Allen, a diabetic, eats ice cream in violation of her dietary exchange protocol. Is eating the ice cream an event or an outcome? Eating ice cream in this case is an event, a discrete behavior, the outcome of which might be added body weight, sugar in her urine, or perhaps even diabetic coma.

3. An article in the local newspaper reported a 25% increase in automobile-related deaths in the past 12 months. Are these deaths events or outcomes? The deaths are outcomes of the individuals' behaviors (events) related to the automobile accidents that took their lives.

4. A group of patients attending a health department clinic have been identified as chronically noncompliant with their high-blood pressure medications. Is this failure to follow a therapeutic regimen an event or an outcome? This question does not have a clear answer. If the instructions on how to comply with the regimen were understood by the patients, then not taking the medications properly would make up a chain of events. If the patients did not understand how to take the medication properly, or did not see the importance of taking it, then the noncompliance would be an outcome. In the latter case, what would be the event(s)? The events would include a chain of behaviors involved with the failure of the health care providers to educate the patients adequately about taking their medication.

The choice of a chain of events or an outcome as the target for an educational program greatly influences the program planning process. Determining whether what we observe in clients are events or outcomes may also be difficult. In looking at health behavior, however, we try to focus on the specific features of the event(s) or outcome(s) that most directly influence(s) health status. Ideally, we would find a key behavior, or a pivotal aspect of a behavior chain, to reinforce or to suppress and thereby influence its frequency of occurrence and prevent a negative outcome from developing.

Predisposing, Enabling, and Reinforcing Factors—the PRECEDE Model

The PRECEDE model is valuable in health education and promotion planning because it provides a format for identifying factors related to health behaviors (Fig. 3–2). PRECEDE is an acronym for "predisposing, reinforcing, and enabling causes in educational diagnosis and evaluation."[19]

Health behavior may be categorized by factors that contribute to its emergence. Three categories of factors are predisposing, enabling, and reinforcing.[19] These three categories of factors form the PRECEDE model, which makes it possible to sort the behaviors that we observe into units for program planning. Through studying a health behavior or outcome, and classifying its dimensions in terms of predisposing, enabling, and / or reinforcing factors, the planning process is simplified.

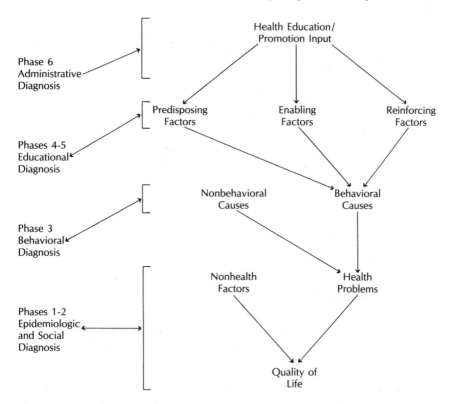

Fig. 3–2. The PRECEDE Model. (Adapted from: Green, L. W., Kreuter, M. W., Deeds, S. G., and Partridge, K. B.: Health, Education Planning: A Diagnostic Approach. Palo Alto, California, Mayfield, 1980, p. 3.)

Predisposing (P) factors are those forces that function to motivate an individual or group to take action. Knowledge, beliefs, attitudes, values, cultural mores and folkways, and genetic heritage all may function as predisposing factors. The key consideration in understanding predisposing factors is the extent to which behavior can be forecast.

Enabling (E) factors include both personal skills and available resources needed to perform a behavior. Enabling factors are those attributes of individuals, groups, and health care delivery systems that make it possible for actions to occur. The key consideration in understanding enabling factors as they relate to health behaviors or outcomes is the extent to which their absence will prevent an action from occurring.

Reinforcing (R) factors provide incentive for health behaviors or outcomes to be maintained. Reinforcement may come from an individual or group, from persons or institutions in the immediate environment, or from society. The key consideration in understanding reinforcing factors is the extent to which their absence would mean a loss of support for current actions of an individual or group.

Classifying health behaviors or outcomes in terms of the factors that predispose their occurrence, provide reinforcement for maintenance and enable their expression, contributes greatly to program planning. Given these data, we can proceed to analyze in depth behaviors or outcomes, and apply our results in the program plan.

The first step in the PRECEDE model is to identify whether factors that contribute to the health behavior in question are in the predisposing, reinforcing, or enabling category. The health professional must then prioritize the factors within and between the categories.

Factors are considered of a priority nature on the basis of their significance in effecting the health behavior in question, the degree to which the factor can be changed, and the resources available to address the particular causative factor(s).[19] Once priority factors are identified, they provide the basis for developing learning objectives. These objectives direct the future action of the program.

Analyzing Events and Outcomes—the SORC Model

How does one go about analyzing in depth a chain of events, a single event, or an outcome as the focus for a community health education program? A useful way to approach this problem is the SORC model.[20] The SORC model analyzes events or outcomes by categorizing the following components: stimulus antecedent variables (S), organism variables (O), response variables (R), and consequences (C).

Stimulus Antecedent (S). These are events in life that prompt us to produce a specific behavior. Health behaviors are the result of our interactions with the environment. In this sense, health behavior can be viewed from an operant conditioning perspective. When we perceive a specific stimulus, we produce a conditioned response. The response produced occurs because of past learning. In previous situations, producing the response resulted in some sort of positive consequence. For example, many overweight people attribute their inability to lose weight to environmental stimuli. They eat almost unconsciously, they report, as a response to nervous tension, television advertising, available food, and many other stimuli. They claim there is no cognitive process involved, that they simply perceive the stimulus (tension, appetizing food) and begin to eat. The act of eating produces a positive short-term consequence in this case; anxiety reduction, reducing "hunger pains," or both.

In considering the health behavior of individuals or groups, it is overly simplistic to look for such obvious stimuli. We know that in our society there are innumerable stimuli that may have application to health practices. In addition, all individuals do not interpret the same stimuli in the same way. For example, if a person says that he is going on a diet, the stimulus for the response may be derived personally (how I look), from important others (my wife says that I'm putting on weight), or from external sources that are related to the society in which we live (television advertising for diet soft drinks). It is likely that the motivation to go on a diet comes from the desire to look better for oneself and others, which arises as a result of various combinations of stimuli. The interpretation of stimuli is highly individualized.

Organism Variables (O). These are the individual differences, due to biologic factors and past learning, that influence our behavior. They are part of our internal functioning, and include our biologic functions, thoughts, and feelings about ourselves, as well as standards for self evaluation. In health education, one of the most perplexing problems we face is how to motivate someone to take preventive action or preserve their health when they have no symptoms of ill health. In such a case, the organism variables include not only the predisposing variables that make one susceptible to developing a disease, but also the processes within the individual that result in denial of susceptibility, leading to the notion that efforts directed toward prevention should not be a high personal priority.

Responses (R). These behaviors (events) may reflect both the intensity of stimuli that precede them and the consequences that follow them. Responses can occur in three overlapping domains: cognitive (verbal), physiologic, and overt motor. In health education, common responses are those associated with avoidance of preventive measures. For example, we might interview a woman and discuss prevention of death from breast cancer through Breast Self Exam (BSE). On the basis of breast cancer, a dreaded consequence, the woman could produce responses in the *cognitive* domain by trying to change the subject away from her vulnerability to breast cancer; or, she could produce a *physiologic* response through involuntarily sweating; or, she could get up and leave, an *overt motor* response to the interview-stimulus that produced the discomfort. The duration, frequency, pervasiveness, and magnitude of the response(s) enable us to gain perspective on how serious the client perceives the stimulus or stimuli to be.

Consequences (C). These are the results of behavior(s). Consequences may be reinforcing and produce an increase in the frequency of the behavior over time; or, they may be repressive, leading to a reduction in the frequency of the behavior. Like any other behavior, health behaviors may be maintained or suppressed by their consequences. From a health education perspective, the long-term consequences from overeating include obesity, and, if continued over time, dangerous circulatory diseases. For the person who overeats, however, the most important consequence, a short-term consequence, may be a release of tension that accompanies eating. In this case, the short-term consequence would help to maintain the overeating behavior despite the negative long-term consequence. A health education program that failed to include treatment for nervous tension would be doomed from the start.

The timing of consequences relative to behaviors is important. The closer the consequence is to the behavior (event) in time, the more powerful is the consequence. Some behaviors have short-term negative consequences and positive consequences in the long term. Exercising may be unpleasant

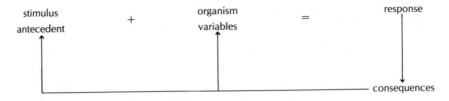

Fig. 3–3. The SORC Model.

to some individuals, by making them hot, sweaty, and tired, for example, but will produce positive consequences over time through weight loss and overall fitness.

Understanding the role of consequences is crucial to understanding health behavior. Consequences may be identified as outcomes, as in the "event and outcome" sense. In most cases, however, the outcomes that we decide to use for program planning—hypertension or heart disease as outcomes to chronic obesity and smoking, for example—are the results of chains of events and outcomes. The outcome that we see as a disease is actually the result of a long series of individual behaviors and the consequences of those behaviors. Each behavior in the chain has its own stimuli and consequences. In these cases, the short-term consequences are not negative at all. It is important to consider the consequences of these individual behaviors in planning health education programs. The frequency of behaviors that are repeated have some sort of positive consequence.

The major benefit of the SORC model (see Fig. 3–3) is that it provides a format for categorizing data that reflect health behaviors and outcomes. The SORC model is equally applicable to groups and individuals. With groups, there is an added dimension to consider—the interactions of group members with one another.

The following example shows how predisposing, enabling, and reinforcing factors are combined with SORC to give a complete definition of the problem for a health education program. In Chapter 2, employees in manufacturing industries were identified as one potential target population. A program may be developed for members of this population to help them avoid occupational injuries.

Predisposing, enabling, and reinforcing factors can be considered as they relate to the incidence of work-related accidental injury. We would identify predisposing factors by studying the target population to determine the level of safety knowledge; their attitudes, values, and beliefs about safety on the job; and their cultural values as they might apply to avoidance of personal risk. Enabling factors would include emphasis on safe conduct from management, availability of equipment to prevent injury, and any other factors that facilitate accident prevention. Factors that reinforce safe and unsafe behaviors would be found in such things as work incentives related to accident-free plants, enforcement of rules requiring use of specified safety devices, and also attitudes of workers toward those persons injured through their own lack of safe behavior.

After consideration of predisposing, enabling, and reinforcing factors, back injuries due to careless lifting practices may be isolated as a target behavior to analyze further. Analysis of the event "lifting heavy objects" can be conducted with the aid of the SORC model.

Stimulus antecedent variables would include the occupational routine that makes lifting a regular task, pressure from oneself to lift an object that is too heavy, and pressure from co-workers. Organism variables would include back strength, knowledge of lifting methods, evaluation of one's own strength, and expectations of oneself about lifting heavy objects. The response is the lifting of the object, with the proper / improper utilization of lifting methods. There are two possible consequences, with separate impacts on the individual. If the object is lifted successfully, with no injury, the consequence is positive. The message to the individual is that there is no need to be concerned about lifting properly. Obviously, this is a dangerous situation. The individual is now in a position that renders him susceptible to injury because he will continue to lift improperly. If the individual lifts the object and experiences back pain of sufficient severity, the message received is quite different.

Using the results of analysis with predisposing, enabling, and reinforcing factors, in addition to an in-depth analysis of the specific behavior using SORC, we are able to select some targets for our health education program. One target might be knowledge, both of proper ways to lift and evaluation of one's own strength; another could be the cultural values of the workers, i.e., manhood being demonstrated through taking risks and proving one's strength.

METHODS FOR COLLECTING DATA ON HEALTH BEHAVIORS AND OUTCOMES

In Chapter 2, several methods to collect information for diagnosing community health problems were discussed. When we need to collect data on *specific* health behaviors for the purpose of program planning there are a variety of methods from which to choose. Three methods—direct observation, self-report, and role playing—are described.

Direct Observation

Direct observation involves observing and recording the occurrences of a defined event, or the unmistakable outcome of the event.[17] The body weight of clients attempting weight loss and plasma cotinine levels in smokers trying to quit are examples of one type of direct observation of outcomes.[21] These measures are commonly referred to as "dependent measures," because the observed values are in some way dependent on the behaviors that preceded them. Body weight reflects caloric intake and exercise; plasma cotinine reflects exposure to nicotine from cigarettes. In health education, the by-products of health behavior are usually much easier to observe directly than are the behaviors themselves.

Direct observation also may be used to collect data on events themselves.[22] Using a predetermined definition for the event and a scheme for recording, an observer monitors interactions and records occurrence of an event. Additional data reflecting the circumstances in which the event occurs may also be recorded. For example, suppose we are planning a patient education program for unwed mothers. The program will emphasize proper maternal nutrition and infant care, and will also seek to enhance the self-esteem of the clients (unwed mothers). In conducting an analysis of the setting in which the program will take place, we are able to diagnose one problem to be a judgmental attitude on the part of the staff. We are told, and see some direct evidence, that some of the staff feel that to be pregnant out of wedlock is sinful, and that the girls in the institution should be ashamed of their behavior. Because this attitude could adversely effect our self-esteem-building activities if perceived by the residents of the institution, we develop a goal statement that includes staff attitudes and behaviors in our program. How can we come to a more complete understanding of the staff attitudes and behaviors, and to the supposed judgmental attitude? We could design a system for direct observation of the staff through which we would define any comment or remark referring to the pregnant state of the residents and their unmarried status in all but official communications as a behavior to record. Through further elaboration of our system, we could also record data on the circumstances under which the target behaviors occurred. If we could collect such data, they would help us to understand more completely the frequency and the circumstances under which the specified behavior occurred. On the basis of these data, we could plan our program to include specific "sensitivity" training for new staff. The process of direct observation would have to be carefully designed in this case because in many circumstances it would be unethical to station a person in the institution to record observations covertly. A solution might be to station an observer to record overtly, with the particular behavior not delineated explicitly. Great care must be taken in these matters to be certain that civil and human rights of persons are not violated.

Self-Report

Self-report measures are designed to provide data for program planning, and also to promote self-awareness in the clients. Self-report is the self-reporting of specified behaviors (events) by subjects.[23-25] A situation is developed wherein the individual records the occurrence of the behaviors and the circumstances in which they occur (see Fig. 3–4). These tactics enable us to collect data on health behaviors without having to observe the client directly. In our example of the home for unwed mothers, we could design

Method 1.

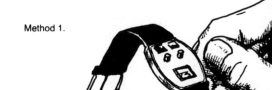

Each time the event of interest occurs it is counted. For example, counting and occurrence of eating between meals gives an estimate of "snacking" behavior.

Method 2.

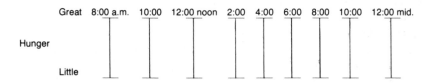

Great 8:00 a.m. 10:00 12:00 noon 2:00 4:00 6:00 8:00 10:00 12:00 mid.

Hunger

Little

"Thermometer" Chart. At the times given, the user of the chart places an "X" on the verticle line. For example, at two hour intervals, record intensity of hunger.

Method 3.

		Type of Food	Amount	Where, When Eaten	How Prepared
Day 1:	Breakfast				
	Lunch				
	Supper				
	Others				
Day 2:	Breakfast				
	Lunch				
	Supper				
	Others				

One type of dietary recall device.

Fig. 3–4. Self-report devices; three methods for recording events.

a simple chart for the staff to record each instance in which they made comments on the pregnancy of a resident in connection with her marital status. These procedures would enable us to obtain a count of the occurrences of the specified behavior, and in addition would make the staff aware of their activities. Through counting, the staff comes to know how often they engage in the specified behavior. Increased self-awareness might reduce the occurrence of the behavior to the point that further attention would not be necessary. On the other hand, through documentation of the circumstances in which the behavior occurred, the health educator might become aware that the behavior is more a reflection of the nature of the job requirements of the staff than of any attitude toward the residents of the home. When the frequency of occurrence of a behavior is reduced as a result of increased awareness produced through direct attention to the behavior, the reduction in behavior is called *reactivity*.[26, 27] Some behaviors can be successfully eliminated through reactivity, but certainly not all. Three methods for self-reporting are illustrated in Figure 3–4.

Role Playing

This activity should be familiar to most health educators.[28, 29] In role playing, clients act out a scene or scenes that depict specific behavioral sequences from their lives. In program planning, we can use role playing to collect valuable data on the interaction among various forces in clients' lives. Role playing is particularly useful in understanding the dynamics of interactions among patients, patients' families, and health providers.[17] In our example of the home for unwed mothers, role playing could help us understand the circumstances in which the staff might discuss the marital status of the pregnant residents. Additionally, we might use role playing to increase the sensitivity of the staff by having them act out their own reactions to the behaviors of the staff if they were residents of the institution. When using role playing, it is important to design the activities carefully. The role playing situations must depict realistic circumstances. The facilitator must know what to look for in the reactions of the players. The ways in which feedback is given also must be planned carefully.

Voluminous literature is available on direct observation, self-report measures, and role playing.[22, 30–32] Additionally, other methods of data collection are available.[33] Combinations of these methods and others, adapted to the particular setting in which they are to be used, allow the collection of data on health behaviors and outcomes. The goal of data collection in this sense is to come to a greater understanding of the target behavior(s) and the circumstances surrounding their occurrence.

ASSESSING EDUCATIONAL READINESS

Defining the events or outcomes completely is a major part of "defining the problem" in program planning. The remaining part of problem definition involves determining the educational readiness of the target population. Educational readiness is the extent to which the target group possesses the prerequisite attitudes, skills, and environmental qualities necessary to learn and use what the program will provide. To plan a health education program

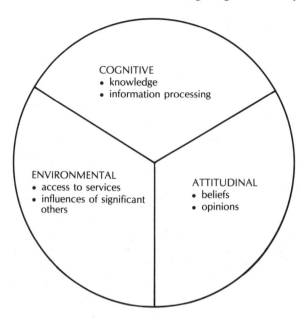

FIG. 3–5. The components of educational readiness.

rationally, we must not only know what issue we wish to confront, but also what tools for learning the members of our target population possess. These tools largely determine the methods from which we can choose to design our educational approach.

Educational readiness can be considered from three different perspectives: cognitive, attitudinal, and environmental (see Fig. 3–5).

Cognitive Factors

The cognitive domain includes knowledge, communication skills, and the ability to process new information internally. A vast array of separate skills and processes is included in the assimilation of new information by a human being. This area of inquiry is rightly the province of the psychologist or psychiatrist, but health educators, as well as other community educators, need to be able to assess the educational skills of their clients. The ability of the client to read and understand health education materials, to remember specific facts, to synthesize related facts and ideas into concepts, and to apply concepts to oneself are basic skills required for learning in the class-room. Community health education programs, however, are not designed solely for classroom teaching. What is needed in assessing cognitive skills for health education programs is information about how well our clients are able to process health education in the settings in which we will interact with them. The skills needed for success in the classroom may not apply as strongly to the community setting.[34] How, then, can the level of cognitive functioning be assessed in view of our needs?

Open communication, taking time to talk with clients, is the best way to address the cognitive aspect of educational readiness for community health education. The way in which clients acquire new information about important aspects of their lives often gives valuable clues to the level of cognitive functioning.[33] If clients acquire new information through reading and research—going to the library and reading "Consumer Reports" about the value of a new product, for example—rather than through the opinions of their friends and acquaintances, then they must be able to read and understand reasonably well to be successful. Furthermore, reading must be an important, useful skill to them. If they rely on mass media exclusively to acquire new information about important aspects of their life, on the other hand, then their reading ability or the importance that they attach to reading may be in question. Opinions about local current events may be formed through many channels, including the editorial page of the local newspaper, or some other written source. Do they know what is the predominant political leaning of the local newspaper(s)? This information may help us to understand better the level of cognitive functioning in our target group and will be invaluable in our efforts to arrive at a conclusion about the cognitive dimension of the educational readiness of our target group. Health knowledge is also considered a part of cognitive functioning. Clients' lack of knowledge about health, disease, and their own bodies may be a cause of their difficulty. An accurate assessment of clients is needed to plan for change.

Attitudinal Factors

Attitudes and beliefs about health-related matters held by the target group are sometimes difficult to assess. While generalized attitudes held in common by the most vocal community residents are often obvious, the private beliefs and opinions of individuals often escape notice unless carefully sought; consequently, it is often challenging to determine the attitudes held by a particular target group of community residents toward a specific health-related issue. As community health educators, we need to know and understand the attitudes that our clients have toward health. Program planners must understand how the target group will view a new health program, or even a revision of an existing program. Along with an understanding of the target population's attitude toward health, program planners need to have a grasp of the attitude toward learning and participation in health programs held by the target population.

Attitudes toward learning vary widely in most communities, particularly among adults.[9] When assessing educational readiness, a definite distinction should be made between attitudes toward *school* and toward *learning*.[34] Few people in our society can achieve any degree of success without learning, but many achieve success without being particularly successful in school. Many adults—and many school-age children—have a negative attitude toward school, which is easily confused with a negative attitude toward learning. For planning community health education programs, a clear picture of the target population's attitude toward acquiring new knowledge is required. That a community or target group has a negative attitude toward the way learning is done in school is an indication of the educational methods least likely to produce the results we want.

Another dimension of attitudinal readiness are attitudes toward health concerns. Many communities have residents with strong feelings about open discussion of human sexual processes, but many other less inflammatory topics may produce equally strong reactions in some target groups. For example, obesity is not universally accepted to mean that one is in poor health. In some cultural groups, what most health professionals would consider a potentially dangerous weight problem is considered a sign of prosperity and good health. Given such a situation, a health education program that ignored the cultural factors favoring being overweight would be doomed to failure. The extent to which a target group can be educated about a particular health problem is in part determined by their attitude toward the seriousness of the problem.

In most community settings, the use of attitudinal inventories to assess attitudinal readiness is largely ineffective. Attitudes toward health concerns can be indirectly assessed by observing the target group. If a particular condition is either rarely seen or very common, the community will most likely not view the condition as a serious problem. Most people adopt a positive attitude toward their current practices. Therefore, if a condition is common and is not obviously causing great harm, there is probably no problem in the eyes of the community. If a health problem is never seen and only rarely experienced, it is also probably not a community concern. If a more formalized assessment of attitudes is needed, several relatively simple methods may be employed.[35, 36]

Environmental Factors

Many environmental factors directly or indirectly influence educational readiness, including access to mass media, family relationships, extended social relationships, socioeconomic status, and local politics. These factors influence educational readiness when they either facilitate or limit the educational process. Suppose a weight control class is planned for a particular target group. Some environmental factors that might affect the program could include the availability of affordable child care, the attitudes of the local culture and particularly the clients' families toward weight control, and the clients' access to a variety of foods. The environment encompassing the clients will largely determine whether they are able to make optimal use of the health education provided. Consideration of the environmental factors in health education is essential.

In assessing educational readiness, an understanding of how the target group is likely to respond to education is needed. This understanding will help in presenting health education so that the clients' cognitive skills and resources are utilized within the boundaries established by their attitudes and the environment in which they live and work.

DETERMINING PROGRAM FOCUS

Health education and promotion programs may focus on individuals, groups, or the entire community. The health professional selects the appropriate level of program focus on the basis of the problem under consideration, the behavior or behaviors related to the problem, the suspected causes of the behavior or behaviors, resources available to address the problem, and the anticipated likelihood of success of the program.

It is essential that the provider of health education and promotion services identify the proper level of focus so that appropriate educational methods can be determined. Some methods of delivering educational messages are more appropriate for the individual than for the group.

Focus on Individuals

Health education and promotion draws from a variety of theoretical perspectives in behavioral science to specify different levels of program focus. A health education and promotion program that focuses on the individual is based on the determination that the individual recipients of the program possess the ability and resources to initiate and maintain the specified behavioral change on their own; one-to-one patient education is a program of this sort. This approach is based on the individual as the learner having the ability to take action on information and skills taught by the provider. Some health promotion programs may also require that the client participate in an individualized risk appraisal with the behavioral change desired being a reduction of health risks on the part of the individual.

Focus on Groups

In group-focused health education and promotion programs, the significance of group interactions and characteristics are the forces that prompt and reinforce behavioral change in individual group members. Weight-loss support groups are an example of the group level of focus. Individual members of the group receive reinforcement and social satisfaction. Some of their social interaction and dependency needs are met through the small group.

Principles of group dynamics are followed when health providers use small groups as a focus of delivering health education and promotion programs. Group dynamics is "the process of interaction of an individual and the group. Group dynamics is concerned with the effect of a group upon an individual's readiness to change or to maintain certain standards or norms."[37]

Family networks, peer groups, and work groups can often influence behavioral change. Methods of delivering health education and promotion to small groups often include continuing education and in-service programs, peer modeling, and disease-oriented support groups. Individuals must feel a part of the group for group education to be successful.

Focus on Communities

Community-focused health education and promotion programs draw on the significance of community identity to bring about positive behavioral change. Much like small groups, a community has a means of reinforcing the individual and regulating the range of change within the community. A community-focused health education and promotion program draws on the strength of the community to address problems and behaviors that are beyond the reach of the individual or small group alone. Community organizing, organizational development, and social marketing are examples of behavioral change strategies focused on the community level.

Community organization includes "those efforts by which groups sharing a common interest are assisted in identifying their specific needs and goals, mobilizing resources within their communities, and in other ways taking action leading to the achievement of the goals they have set collectively."[38] Organizational development is "the application of a long-range, planned change technology designed to improve the problem-solving and renewal process by which an organization changes its culture."[39] Social marketing is "the design, implementation, and control of program seeking to increase the acceptability of a social idea or cause in a target group(s)."[40]

Each of these strategies focuses on bringing about change in large organizations or the entire community. Such strategies utilize the functions and interactions of large systems or communities as the means to solve or address health problems.

The following example incorporates various models of behavioral and educational analysis as applied to an individual.

Example 1. The Case of Mrs. R.

Mrs. R. is a 45-year-old woman, 64 inches tall, 200 pounds, with essential hypertension controlled by medication. She was referred to the health educator by a physician, who saw her regularly in the health department outpatient clinic. She was referred to the health educator specifically to lose weight.

At the initial intake interview, the health educator concentrated on establishing rapport with Mrs. R. while learning about her lifestyle in general, and her eating habits and exercise in particular. Several important things quickly came to light. First, Mrs. R. and her family (husband and son) were a low-income family, and could not afford to buy food in much variety. Second, Mrs. R.'s husband was described by her as a "picky eater," and would not eat any vegetables except potatoes and squash. The only way he would eat these vegetables was if they were fried in lard. The remainder of the family diet consisted of fried hamburger, chicken occasionally (also fried), and other convenience foods such as hot dogs. Third, Mrs. R. stated that she had "always had" a weight problem, and had been significantly overweight since about age 13 years. She had gone on diets in the past, and had successfully lost up to 40 pounds, but always gained the weight back. Mrs. R. stated that she wanted to lose weight, but felt anxious about having a goal set for her that would be too high.

Name:		Age:	Sex:	Date:
Referred by/from:		Education:		

1. Behavior during interview and physical description:

2. Presenting problem:
   A. Relevant history:

   B. Current status:

   C. Consequences of problem:

3. Other related situations or problems:

4. Educational readiness: (cognitive skills, attitude, environment)

5. Recommended educational goals, objectives:

6. Prognosis:

7. Referral/consultation recommended:

Intake interviewer:

Fig. 3-6.   Intake interview format.

At the conclusion of the intake interview (see Fig. 3–6), the health educator developed a self-report schedule for Mrs. R. to complete at home during the week until her next appointment. She was to bring the completed report with her for the next appointment with the health educator. The self-report schedule is shown in Figure 3–7. In addition to the self-report schedule, the health educator personally weighed Mrs. R. and plotted her weight on a chart. The health educator then showed the chart to Mrs. R. and explained that the chart would be used to keep track of her progress, and that she would be weighed every visit (see Fig. 3–8).

When Mrs. R. was next seen, her self-report schedule was not completed sufficiently to allow for any hypotheses or conclusions to be drawn. The health educator praised Mrs. R. for completing as much as she had of the schedule, and explained the importance of getting to know what her everyday diet was like. The health educator continued to explore other topics with Mrs. R. and through the course of the conversation began to feel that one of the primary difficulties Mrs. R. was having with her eating habits was related to her husband's working schedule. Mrs. R.'s husband worked so that he left home about 2:00 p.m. daily and returned after 11:00 p.m. The family ate a "normal" breakfast meal, a "lunch" meal before Mr. R. went to work, and then Mrs. R. and her son had

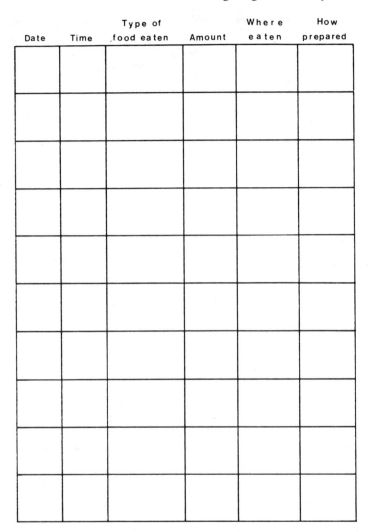

Date	Time	Type of food eaten	Amount	Where eaten	How prepared

Fig. 3–7. Self-report schedule for dietary recall.

supper at about 6:00 p.m. When Mr. R. returned home from work he was in the habit of eating a large meal. At his request Mrs. R. would share this meal with him, although she had already eaten three meals, plus snacks, during the day. Upon realizing this sequence of events, the health educator explained to Mrs. R. that she could not possibly lose the desired weight with the number of calories currently consumed and her exercise level. Mrs. R. responded that her husband felt very strongly about having an evening meal with his wife, and she doubted her ability to convince him that she needed to change her habits. The health educator assigned Mrs. R. to continue completing her self-report schedule, and added a category of "foods eaten after 11:00 p.m."

At the next meeting with the health educator Mrs. R. produced a virtually complete self-report schedule. The report showed that Mrs. R. was eating her heaviest meal just before retiring for the night. In addition, the foods eaten by Mrs. R. at her 11:00 p.m. meal were almost exclusively fried. At this meeting, Mrs. R. was weighed and had lost 2 pounds. She was disappointed with the small amount of weight loss, but the health educator attempted to buoy her spirits by pointing out that weight loss does not come quickly.

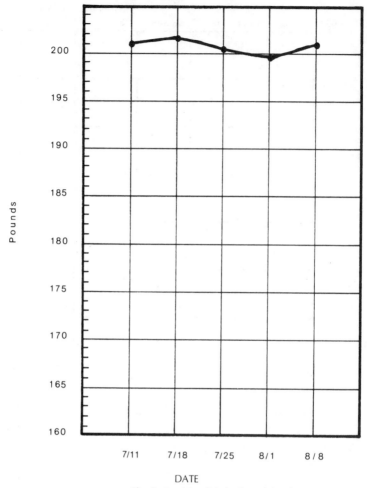

DATE

Fig. 3–8.   Mrs. R.'s body weight chart.

The self-report schedule and the interviews with Mrs. R. enabled the health educator to assess Mrs. R.'s educational readiness informally. Her self-report schedule showed that Mrs. R. was literate, and the interviews showed that she was able to conceptualize, at least where nutrition and weight loss were concerned. Mrs. R.'s attitude toward changing her eating behaviors was positive, but her environment was a source of concern. The health educator suspected that Mrs. R.'s husband was not really supportive of his wife's weight loss efforts, and that this concern would have to be explored further. Based on the self-report schedule results and the educational assessment, the following behaviors were identified as targets for change.

1. Late night eating. Mrs. R. should either eliminate this meal entirely, or substitute foods with less calories.
2. Cooking practices. Mrs. R. should stop frying everything she eats. She should substitute boiled vegetables at a minimum.
3. Snacking. Mrs. R. needs to eliminate between-meal eating.

Mrs. R. reacted favorably to changing the behaviors identified by the health educator. She did express concern with any added cost to her food budget, and also seemed unenthusiastic about preparing her own food separately from the rest of the family. She felt that she would not be able to induce her husband to modify his eating habits, but understood that frying foods in lard was adding excess calories to her diet.

In summary, the analysis of Mrs. R.'s current lifestyle relative to her weight problem suggested the following as factors helping to maintain her current behaviors.

1. Predisposing—metabolic rate, husband's work schedule and dominance in decisions about family eating habits, limited repertoire of cooking methods.
2. Enabling—husband's attitude toward Mrs. R.'s weight control efforts, eating habits, limited variety of foods, limited food budget.
3. Reinforcing—no negative social consequences for overweight, no exacerbation of hypertension due to overweight, family support for current physical condition.

Analysis using the SORC variables suggested the following as factors helping to maintain Mrs. R.'s current behaviors.

S—feelings of hunger, available food, daily schedule, husband's request.

O—caloric intake in excess of physiologic needs, appestat, lack of overt physical distress related to diet.

R—eating excess calories.

C—positive: husband's satisfaction with Mrs. R.'s behavior, satisfaction of feelings of hunger, anxiety reduction.

negative: weight gain, lack of reinforcement from health educator.

Example 2. Inhaled Crop Sprays Among Farmers

After several discussions with local physicians, community health officials became aware of a potential serious health problem among the farm population of the county. Improper use of crop sprays and dusts was resulting in increasing incidence of several diseases. The health educator at the county health department was assigned to develop a health education program, and was to work with the county agricultural extension agent. The first problem faced by the health educator was how to determine the behaviors to deal with in a health education program. The following system for behavioral analysis was developed.

1. The health educator and the agricultural extension agent would identify farm study units. A farm study unit would be defined as all persons living or working on a farm. Individuals who worked on the farm infrequently, such as inspectors, would not be included. This identification would include all socioeconomic strata and all types of farm workers.
2. After identifying the farm study units, the health educator and the agriculture extension agent would interview a "representative sample" of those identified, and become familiar with their individual practices in general in handling crop sprays and dusts. To make the interviewer more systematic, role-playing situations would be developed in which the farm units would demonstrate specific procedures in using crop sprays and dusts. An observation checklist of behaviors would be developed to record interview and role-playing data (see Fig. 3–9).
3. On the basis of the results of the interviews and the observations of role playing, the health educator would determine behaviors to be the focus of the health education program.

Using these procedures, the following occurred.

1. Ten farms were identified as representing typical farms in the county. All of the farms were "family farms," but most had supplemental workers employed most of the time. Thus, the target population included not only the farm families themselves, but also the farmhands.
2. Because only 10 farms were involved, all persons associated with these 10 farms were interviewed. The agriculture extension agent and the health educator decided to work as a team in the interviews, because after testing the interview procedures, neither felt comfortable assessing health risks out of their own area of expertise. The role-playing exercises were the most difficult part of the interviews to conduct, but were also the most valuable. In most of the interviews, the subjects hesitated about the role-playing concept, but use of the structured role-playing protocol enabled the interviewer to conduct the assessment.
3. The following behaviors were identified for use in the health education program.
   a. use of protective devices: clothing, masks.
   b. proper use of spraying equipment, including care of the equipment.
   c. exposure of others not directly involved with spraying
   d. timing crop spraying with climate, weather.

1. Date: _____
2. Farm study unit: _____
   a. List individuals by age and sex: _____
3. Crops grown: _____
   a. Spray (type and how used): _____

4. Role-playing checklist.

	Acceptable	Not Acceptable	Comments
a. Equipment Maintenance	_____	_____	_____
b. Protective Clothing	_____	_____	_____
1. mask or respirator	_____	_____	_____
2. eye protection	_____	_____	_____
c. Equipment Use			
1. follows directions for substance	_____	_____	_____
2. accounts for climate	_____	_____	_____
3. accounts for weather	_____	_____	_____
d. Protection of others	_____	_____	_____

5. Analysis (tentative ideas about maintenance of current behaviors)

	Comments
a.1. Predisposing factors:	_____
2. Enabling factors:	_____
3. Reinforcing factors:	_____
b.1. Stimulus antecedents:	_____
2. Organism variables:	_____
3. Responses:	_____
4. Consequences:	_____

Fig. 3–9. Interview / Observation Checklist

The examples of Mrs. R. and of the farm population identified practices that led to unhealthy conditions. In planning community health education programs, an understanding of factors that contribute to the initiation and maintenance of these practices is essential. The anticipated outcome of a community health education program would be to alter contributing factors resulting in behavioral change.

REFERENCES

1. Bedworth, D.A., and Bedworth, A.E.: Health Education: A Process for Human Effectiveness. New York, Harper & Row, 1978.
2. Dubos, R.: Man Adapting. New Haven, Yale University Press, 1965.

3. Burbach, H.J., and Decker, L.E.: A growing imperative. *In* Planning and Assessment in Community Education. Edited by H.J. Burbach and L.E. Decker. Midland, Michigan, Pendell, 1977.
4. Rossi, P.H., Freeman, H.E., and Wright, S.R.: Evaluation: A Systematic Approach. Beverly Hills, Sage, 1979.
5. Fodor, J.T., and Dalis, G.T.: Health Instruction: Theory and Application. 3rd Ed. Philadelphia, Lea & Febiger, 1981.
6. Weiss, C.H.: Evaluation Research: Methods of Assessing Program Effectiveness. Englewood Cliffs, New Jersey, Prentice-Hall, 1972.
7. Kazdin, A.E.: Behavior Modification in Applied Settings. Homewood, Illinois, Dorsey Press, 1975.
8. Wolf, M.M.: Social validity: the case for subjective measurement or how applied behavior analysis is finding its heart. J. Appl. Behav. Anal., *11*(2):203, 1978.
9. Aronson, E.: The Social Animal. 2nd Ed. San Francisco, W.H. Freeman, 1976.
10. Kanfer, F.H., and Grimm, L.G.: Behavioral analysis: selecting target behaviors in the interview. Behav. Modif., *1*:7, 1977.
11. Thorp, R., and Wetzel, R.: Behavior Modification in the Natural Environment. New York, Academic Press, 1969.
12. McFall, R.M.: Behavioral training: a skill acquisition approach to clinical problems. *In* Behavioral Approaches to Therapy. Edited by J.T. Spence, R.C. Carson, and J.W. Thibaut. Morristown, New Jersey, General Learning Press, 1976.
13. Lanyon, R.I., and Lanyon, B.P.: Behavior Therapy: A Clinical Introduction. Reading, Massachusetts, Addison-Wesley, 1978.
14. American Psychiatric Association Task Force on Nomenclature and Statistics: DSM-III; Diagnostic Criteria Draft, New York, American Psychiatric Association, 1978.
15. Ciminero, A.R., Calhoun, K.S., and Adams, H.E., (eds): Handbook of Behavioral Assessment. New York, Wiley, 1977.
16. Peterson, D.R.: The Clinical Study of Social Behavior. New York, Appleton-Century-Crofts, 1968.
17. Rose, S.D.: A Casebook in Group Therapy: A Behavioral Cognitive Approach. Englewood Cliffs, New Jersey, Prentice-Hall, 1980.
18. Miller, L.K.: Principles of Everyday Behavior Analysis. Monterey, California, Brooks-Cole, 1975.
19. Green, L.W., Kreuter, M.W., Deeds, S.G., and Partridge, K.B.: Health Education Planning: A Diagnostic Approach. Palo Alto, California, Mayfield, 1980.
20. Goldfried, M.R., and Sprafkin, J.N.: Behavioral Personality Assessment. Morristown, New Jersey, General Learning Press, 1974.
21. Williams, C.L., Eng, A., Botvin, G.J., Hill, P., and Wynder, E.L.: Validation of students' self-reported cigarette smoking status with plasma cotinine levels. Am. J. Public Health, *69*(12):1272, 1979.
22. Haynes, S.N.: Principles of Behavioral Assessment. New York, Gardner Press, 1978.
23. Kazdin, A.E.: Self-monitoring and behavior change. *In* Self-Control: Power to the Person. Edited by M.J. Mahoney and C.E. Thoresen. Monterey, California, Brooks-Cole, 1974.
24. Lick, J.R., and Katkin, E.S.: Assessment of anxiety and fear. *In* Behavioral Assessment: A Practical Handbook. Edited by M. Hersen and A.S. Bellack. New York, Pergamon, 1976.

25. Walls, R.T., Werner, T.J., Bacon, A., and Zane, T.: Behavior checklists. *In* Behavioral Assessment: New Directions in Clinical Psychology. Edited by J.D. Cone and R.P. Hawkins, New York, Brunner/Mazel, 1977.
26. Lipinski, D.P., and Nelson, R.O.: The reactivity and unreliability of self recording. J. Consult. Clin. Psychol., *42*:119, 1974.
27. McFall, R.M.: Effects of self monitoring on normal smoking behavior. J. Abnorm. Psychol., *35*(2):135, 1970.
28. Read, D.A., and Greene, W.H.: Creative Teaching in Health. 3rd Ed. New York, Macmillan, 1980.
29. Simon, S.B., Howe, L.W., and Kirschenbaum, H.: Values Clarification: A Handbook of Practical Strategies for Teachers and Students. New York, Hart, 1972.
30. Cone, J.D., and Hawkins, R.P., (eds): New Directions in Clinical Psychology. New York, Brunner/Mazel, 1977.
31. Hersen, M., and Bellack, A.S.: Behavioral Assessment: A Practical Handbook. New York, Pergamon, 1976.
32. Nelson, R.O., and Hayes, S.C.: Some current dimensions of behavioral assessment. Behav. Assess. *1*:257, 1979.
33. Webb, E.J., Campbell, D.T., Schwartz, R.D., and Sechrest, L.: Unobtrusive Measures. Chicago, Rand McNally, 1966.
34. Houle, C.O.: The Design of Education. San Francisco, Jossey-Bass, 1972.
35. Reeder, L.G., Ramacher, L.G., and Gorelnik, S.: Handbook of Scales and Indices of Health Behavior. Pacific Palisades, California, Goodyear, 1976.
36. Vincent, R.J.: New scale for measuring attitudes. School Health Rev. *5*(2):19, 1974.
37. Bates, I., and Winder, A.E.: Introduction to Health Education. Palo Alto, California, Mayfield, 1984.
38. Minkler, M.: Ethical issues in community organization. *In* SOPHE Heritage Collection of Health Education Monographs. Vol. 2. Edited by Betty P. Mathews. Oakland, California, Third Party, 1982.
39. Mico, P.R., and Ross, H.: Health Education and Behavioral Science. Oakland, California, Third Party, 1975.
40. Kotler, P.R.: Social marketing. *In* Marketing for Nonprofit Organizations. 2nd Ed. Englewood Cliffs, New Jersey, Prentice-Hall, 1982.

4

Developing a Program Plan

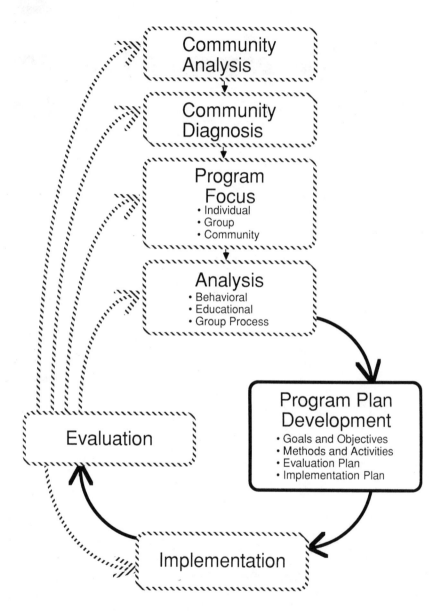

The Health Education / Promotion Planning Model.

4

Developing a Program Plan

In Chapters 1 through 3, we discussed the basis for program planning, described the procedures for community analysis and diagnosis, and presented methods that can be used for analysis of behavior. In this chapter, we apply the information previously presented to the production of a program plan.

Like a blueprint for a house, a progam plan—a "blueprint" for a health education or health promotion program—is critical because the plan provides a guide for the development and implementation of the program. The importance of the plan becomes apparent when its impact on the cycle of planning is considered. As part of the cycle, the program plan sets the agenda for implementation and evaluation. More importantly, it specifies the goals for the program and how those goals will be reached.[1-7]

COMPONENTS OF PROGRAM PLANS

Plans for health education programs typically include many different components. The purpose of programs may differ, but several basic components appear in most cases. The essential components are presented and defined in Table 4–1.

THE PLANNING PROCESS

The process of developing program plans includes several steps that are connected in complex ways (Fig. 4–1). The complicated nature of these connections often makes planning a group effort. Thus, the *first* step in planning is to formulate a group to take on the task. The *second* step is to develop goals, in light of the results of community analysis. The planning group must also be certain that the targets of the program are consulted about the goals. The objectives for the program are developed in the *third*

Table 4–1. Essential Components of Program Plans

Program Plan Components[8, 9]	Definition
Statements of goals	Broad statements that define what the health education program is expected to accomplish
Objectives	Statements that map out the tasks needed to reach a goal, including time frame, direction, and magnitude and measurement of change.
Methods and activities	Means through which the changes will be made. Methods identify the vehicle for education, such as mass media and personal instruction, activities describe the specific ways that education will be applied.
Resources and constraints	Specific resources in the target community that may be used for the program to bring about change. Constraints are forces that are expected to work against the program.
Evaluation plan	Procedures for determining whether the program performed as planned.
Implementation plan	Procedures for introducing the program to the target group.

step of the planning process. Once objectives are developed, resources and constraints are explored in step *four.* Resources may exist in many forms, such as funding, volunteers from the target community, or audiovisual production expertise. Resources are helpful in putting the program into action. Constraints are forces that work against the program. By using the objectives, resources, and constraints, the methods and activities used to reach the program goals can be selected in the *fifth* step. Planning for evaluation and implementation are the *sixth* and *seventh* steps. Competent planning involves consideration of how the program will operate (implementation) and how success or failure will be judged (evaluation) throughout the planning process.

Developing a Working Planning Group

Development of the components of a program plan requires significant effort. As a result, planning usually involves groups of planners rather than

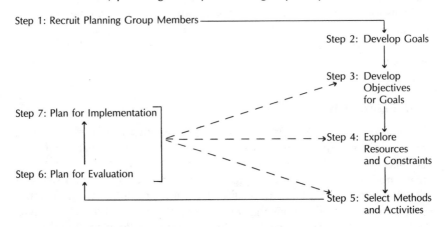

Fig. 4–1. Evaluation and implementation reflect the clarity of objectives, accuracy of estimates of resources and constraints, and the appropriateness of methods and activities.

individuals acting alone. A planning group has the obvious advantage of smaller work loads for each individual. In addition, however, groups provide the potential for incorporating different points of view into the planning process. In planning health education, a diversity of viewpoints is usually valuable.

Recruitment

One key health professional, a health educator, nurse, nutritionist, or physician, often determines the strategies for assembling the planning group, but in some cases the makeup of the group may be dictated by agency policy or rules set down by a funding source. One strategy for assembling a planning group is for those individuals involved in the community analysis and behavioral analysis to appoint the members of the planning group, or to serve themselves. The health professional may, on the other hand, appoint all members of the planning group. In rare but ideal cases, representatives from the target group may be recruited and constitute the planning group. The most essential prerequisites for membership on a planning group are interest in the problems of the target population, willingness to work with other group members, reasonable communication skills, and dependability.

Planning group members can also be recruited through democratic processes. Constituent groups who will receive program services may select representatives to participate in program planning. Caution must be exercised in interpreting the results of selection processes in unknown groups, however, because the same forces that provide for visibility of group members as volunteers may also influence the outcome of other processes.

One very important consideration in selecting a planning group is the inclusion of representatives from the target group. The inclusion of representatives of the target population in the planning process is distinctly advantageous. When members of the target group participate actively in the planning process, there is a feeling of ownership of the program being planned, which facilitates implementation of the program and encourages participation.[9]

Occasionally entire target groups participate in program planning; however, in these instances, the target populations are small and must be homogenous in terms of educational level, degree of motivation toward solving the problem under consideration, and philosophy (how they see themselves in the world).[8, 10]

Individuals often volunteer to serve as members of the planning group; however, when those individuals have personal reasons for promoting the program, they add uncertainty to the planning process and may bias the program that is implemented.[9, 11, 12] The efforts put into program planning by a member or members of the planning group who may have hidden agendas of unspoken goals for the planning process or the program itself may be misdirected and ultimately may influence the success of the program. For example, a community resident serving on a health department advisory council may rather support a community-sponsored health center than a health department outreach program because the resident may perceive he or she has more control over services to be offered.

Identifying and resolving hidden agendas of individual planning group members will reduce the number of obstacles confronted in developing a successful program plan, although such issues may be difficult to resolve. Identification of hidden agendas may be approached through use of key informants or the planning group members themselves, or through group process exercises with the entire planning group. Once any existing hidden agendas are resolved, the group can more readily agree upon common goals for the program and the procedures they will use to develop the program plan.

In selecting representatives of the target group for the planning group, it is easiest to select the most visible persons, that is, those with whom contact has been made most often or those who are the group leaders. That members of a target population are visible does not assure that they are able to represent the view of the whole. Organizers of program plans should be wary of an inclination to favor, consciously or unconsciously, those persons from the target group that may be most friendly or most vocal. No matter who serves on the planning group, the thoughts and needs of the target group must be represented.

In selecting planning group members, it is essential to recruit those persons who can communicate the felt needs of the target group to other members of the planning group. Planning group members representing the target group should be familiar with the patterns of living and the beliefs related to health practices of the target group to the extent that they will be able to provide insight into probable reactions to community health education efforts. In this way, the methods and activities for directing behavior change will be appropriate for the target group.

Orientation to the Task of Planning

The first step in mobilizing the planning group is to orient the group to the process of planning a health education program.[1] Because planning groups, especially those in which members of the target group participate, may be uneven in the extent of members' familiarity with the program planning process, the first task is to acquaint all planning group members with the functioning of a community health education and promotion program and the procedures to be used in developing plans.

The planning group members must begin with a basic understanding of planning. They also must know that the outcome of their efforts will be a health education program designed to meet identified needs of the target group. In some cases, group members may require extensive briefing about how the planning is to be done; pertinent customs and behaviors of the target group (if identified); and federal, state, or local laws that may impact on the planning process. When each member sufficiently understands the tasks, a list of roles needed in the planning process should be developed.

Role Negotiation

During orientation, each group member should come to understand how the planning task ahead relates to his or her own area of expertise. Each group member should be asked to identify where his or her skills or knowledge best fit in with the overall planning process. Each person should understand that he or she has a unique contribution to make. After a list of tasks and the skills required to conduct the program planning tasks is tabulated, initial roles for the group members involved in the planning process can be negotiated. Roles present in a group are often as varied as the individuals constituting the group. Ultimately, the roles needed within the planning group are determined by the nature of the task. A list of roles that may be found within planning groups could include: chairperson, recorder, treasurer, facilitator, summarizer, writer, researcher, agency representative, or target group representative.

Role negotiation may be a threatening process for individuals within the planning group, especially when members of the target group are involved. It is unlikely that target group representatives can be identified with titles such as "community health educator," "public health nurse," or "clergyman." The lack of concise recognition may result in a feeling of alienation. Each group member must feel that he or she has a role that is recognized and valued by the entire group.

Delegation of Responsibility

Up to this point, one or two individuals may have carried the primary responsibility for initiating and overseeing all activities related to the program planning process. These people may have worked alone or acted as a participant in the community analysis as well as conducted the behavioral analysis. He or she may have been instrumental in identifying and recruiting members of the planning group and orienting them to the task at hand. When roles for the planning group are negotiated, however, the health educator could likely end up in a very different role. It is at this point that each member of the planning group should be encouraged to assume responsibility for the program. Each group member must decide what role is appropriate for himself or herself and negotiate with other members of the planning group. The health professional will continue to be involved until the program is self-supporting within the target population; is proven successful, its mission accomplished, and is no longer needed; or is considered unsuccessful and must be discontinued or revised.

The group at this point is ready to act. The results of the community and behavioral analyses must be briefly re-examined and reconfirmed.

Formulating Goals

Goals are statements that describe, in broad terms, what is to be accomplished. Two types of goals to be formulated are those for the program as a whole and those for educational services that will be delivered as part of the program. Even though program goals usually imply goals for education, goals for education must be stated clearly to establish the role of education in reaching program goals.

Program Goals

Program goal statements are intended to communicate intended achievements of the program. Such statements may identify components of the program and the types of services to be included, but usually program goals do not provide a description of the services. Thus, separate statements are needed to establish the goals of the various services. The subsequent discussion is limited to goals for health education and promotion.

Goals for Health Education and Promotion

Goal statements for health education and promotion are broad statements that define what health education should accomplish.[4, 6] Deriving educational goal statements is perhaps the first activity undertaken by the planning group that is specifically related to the final planning document, the health education plan. Because educational goals are the basis for the rest of the planning process, it is essential that they be stated in precise language so that all members of the health education planning group thoroughly understand the exact intention of the statements.

Group process should be used in constructing the educational goal statements. Consensus should be achieved without reservation.[1] Disagreements may occur among planning group members as educational goals are defined. The group leader(s) must exercise care in understanding the nature of each disagreement and its resolution. If consensus related to goals for the educational program cannot be reached, the nature of the planning task should be re-examined, the composition of the planning group should be questioned, and a solution for the dilemma should be decided before any further activities take place. At this stage in planning, evidence of hidden agendas may surface. Formulation of goals provides the first true orientation for the planning process, which often gives rise to a perceived need to shape the future.

Goals provide the framework for program planning; consequently, it is important that they reflect reality in terms of the target population. One of the most common criticisms of health education programs is that they are predicated on the biases of the professionals who deliver the services—whether appropriate or not. Community health education programs are community-based programs, designed to meet needs of the target population. The fact that the community health education programs also serve the needs of the health educators is a by-product only. Goals for education need to reflect the "state of the art" in community health education (health educators should not promise what probably cannot be delivered), but health professionals must be aware that new approaches to solving problems are rarely developed when challenge is avoided.

Statements of Educational Goals

As presented in Chapter 3, two types of educational goal statements are most commonly seen in health education program plans. One is a statement of effect of the educational program on the *client*. The other is a statement of effect of the educational program on the *agency* delivering services to the client. In health education programs directed toward effects on the client, the goals are often stated in terms of *health status changes*. For example, "reducing mortality from cardiovascular diseases by altering the knowledge level, behaviors, and attitudes of the target population regarding blood pressure screening and the dangers of heart disease" is a health status goal.[13] Goals for the educational program may also identify anticipated *changes in behaviors* of the target group members. These behaviors are related to health status. "A reduction in smoking cigarettes" is an example of a goal that specifies behavior change that relates to health status.

In health education programs directed toward changes in the agency, goal statements are often stated in terms of *collective behavioral changes* among staff members; for example, "the staff of the Crescent County Health Department will include planned health education in their duties where appropriate." As stated, this goal statement indicates behavioral change in staff members. This change represents the impact of the health education program on the agency. When programs are designed to effect changes in agencies, there are really two target populations, the clients of the agency and the providers working in the agency itself. By choosing to direct attention toward achieving behavior change in providers, we assume that the clients of the agency will be served. Such an assumption decreases the likelihood of achieving desirable changes in the target population and should be avoided if possible.

Distinguishing between Long- and Short-Term Goals

It may be difficult to distinguish between goals that need to be accomplished soon and goals that are more timeless. For example, a goal of protecting a community against a specific communicable disease such as rubella, which is susceptible to immunization, is clear. It is a short-term goal and can be easily stated in behavioral terms. On the other hand, a goal of improving the health status of people in general is timeless and has no easily identified means of accomplishment in the short term. Thus, it is a long-term goal. Providing health care services involves short-term goal statements that, if successful, should have impact on the more long-term goal of improving health status. Planning groups can easily get snarled in such questions as whether to emphasize long- or short-term goals in planning. When members of the target group participate in program planning, they are likely to object to long-term goals that may seem nebulous in favor of goals that are more action-oriented. The target group may be impatient, wanting immediate and significant outcomes with minimal input. They may not understand the complexity of the behavior change process promoted through the health education program. Through negotiation and communication, the health educator must assist the planning group in understanding the long-range outcomes of the health education program.

In the analysis of Crescent County (see Chapter 2), those persons employed in manufacturing industries were identified as a potential target population. A behavioral analysis of this population (see Chapter 3) revealed that improper lifting techniques, resulting in back injuries, were related to knowledge of proper lifting methods, faulty evaluation of one's strength, and worker values that encourage risk-taking. Based on these factors, the following goals for *education* could be established: (1) workers will learn to avoid back injuries through knowledge of proper techniques for lifting heavy objects, (2) workers will learn to evaluate their own back strength, and (3) workers will learn about the dangers to health, loss of function, and other difficulties resultant from back injuries.

Verifying Educational Goals

Educational goal statements need to be verified by the target population and the program sponsors. Educational goals provide the framework for the rest of the program and dictate program objectives. For this reason, the goals must reflect a realistic solution to the problems of the target population in terms of change that is desirable as well as feasible. The program sponsors are also important in verifying educational goals, for they will ultimately provide support for the program. A firm commitment and agreement with the goals of education from the sponsors of the program provide assurance of support before the time-consuming process of formulating objectives begins. If the target population or the sponsors disagree with the educational goals of the program, it is a simpler task to revise the goal statements than to revise program objectives.

Specifying Objectives

Objectives are precise statements that map out the tasks necessary to reach a goal.[2] They are intended to specify behavior changes needed to achieve a goal. Objectives should be stated clearly in terms of (1) the time frame within which an activity takes place; (2) the direction of change facilitated in the target population, whether client or agency; (3) the magnitude of anticipated change; and (4) a precise definition of the way change is measured.

Generally speaking, objectives are statements composed of two parts, *content* and *behavior*.[2] The content part of the objective identifies the subject matter and the setting, for example, " . . . patients with diabetes coming to the outpatient clinic for periodic maintenance care." The behavior part of the objective spells out what action will be seen in the client as a result of interaction with the activities that you provide in the program, for example, " . . . can interpret the food exchange charts. . . ." Objectives must identify who will be involved in the program; what they will do, stated in behavioral terms; when the action will occur; where the action will occur; and the extent of the behavioral change or action.

Like educational goal statements, once written, objectives must be verified in terms of the target group. If members of the target group participate in the planning group, this process of verification is facilitated. Regardless, objectives must be appropriate for the target population's resources and constraints.

Determining the Time Frame

Time, as an element of objectives, fits into program evaluation particularly well. Time, stated in various terms, is one of the most common evaluative criteria. For example, time may be stated in terms of hours, days, months, or years. Specifying when an activity will be accomplished such as "by the end of 2 months," and for what duration is an important feature of well-written objectives. Great care must be taken when producing program objectives with time parameters because the program may become unduly inhibited by unreasonable time limitations. All activities require lead time to become operational. Lead time is the time required for organization between planning and implementation. When objectives are properly constructed, adequate lead time is included, while pressure is simultaneously exerted to ensure that services are delivered within a predetermined time period.

Specifying Direction of Change

It is assumed that the behavior change specified in the goals and objectives will lead to positive health outcomes. Program objectives that accurately specify behavior change indicators greatly facilitate evaluation. More importantly, specifying the direction of change guides the planning group in determining the content of the health education program; for example, *increasing* the number of times per week an individual exercises or *reducing* the number of between-meal snacks a person eats will lead toward more positive health outcomes. Health educators often err by concentrating on behavioral outcomes of education rather than on the series of educational interventions leading to behavioral outcomes. For health education programs to be successful in achieving behavior change among clients, objectives must be formulated that incorporate series of changes that culminate in an overall behavioral outcome.[14]

Determining the Magnitude of Anticipated Change

Objectives help to spell out how much change is anticipated within a given time period. For example, "within 6 months there will be a 60% reduction in the number of cigarettes smoked." Baseline information that identifies levels of behavior, such as the number of cigarettes smoked per day when the program began, may be of use to the program planner.[14] Perhaps the most important factor in determining the magnitude of anticipated change, however, is the intended target population of the program being planned. How similar or different is this target population from those of similar programs? What results were achieved? How badly does the target population want to change? What differences within the target population are likely to result in resistance to program efforts? Information from the community and behavioral analyses as well as familiarity with the target group will give the planning group some indication of the answers to these questions.

Determining How Change is Measured

The phrase "the way change is measured" is intended to mean a unit of measurement. Effective program objectives should include discrete and fully specified procedures for measuring the effects of the interventions planned for the program.[15] The measure of body weight can be either pounds or kilograms, but the concept is established when the notion of "how much do you weigh" is connected to a single unit of measurement that may be used to compare individuals. In community health education programs, establishing a measure serves to facilitate evaluation, both during and at the conclusion of a program. In addition, a measure describing a complex health education process may help in explaining program activities to agency administrators.

Changes in knowledge can be measured through individual questions on pretests and post-tests, self-reporting, structured interviews, or self-instructional materials. Attitudinal changes are often measured by using similar means. Behavioral changes can be measured by identifying the individual behaviors to be monitored and designing a means of measuring the change. Direct observation, self-reporting, and reports from significant others are often used to measure behavioral changes. (Problems such as these are discussed in Chapter 6.)

In developing objectives, consideration of several key characteristics of effective objectives will help assure success.[2, 16] The planning group must develop objectives that clearly describe content and behavior, are appropriate for the particular target group, are stated in precise behavioral terms, and are measurable (see Fig. 4–2).

Appropriateness. Objectives for community health education programs are most appropriate when they are carefully matched to the needs, customs, values, view of the world, and interests of the target population that were

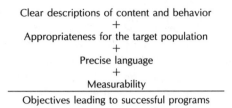

Clear descriptions of content and behavior
+
Appropriateness for the target population
+
Precise language
+
Measurability
_____
Objectives leading to successful programs

Fig. 4–2. A formula for effective objectives.

identified in the community and behavioral analyses. For example, for pregnant teenagers to understand the details of the function of HCTH (human chorionotropic hormone) would be a laudable objective for a prenatal education class, but it would probably be difficult to achieve and of questionable value. It might be more useful if the pregnant teenagers could "list and describe three presumptive signs of pregnancy." Levels of education, cultural background, socioeconomic status, and religiosity are among the factors that influence how well the target population can be expected to accept health education programs. The success of the program hinges on the extent to which the objectives match the needs of the client.

Precision. Although a high level of precision with objectives for community health education programs is difficult to achieve, it is essential to be as precise as possible. One way to be more precise in stating objectives is to choose the behavioral descriptors very carefully (Table 4–2). As discussed in Chapter 3, when selecting descriptors, strive to choose either a behavior or behaviors that can be readily observed, or a behavior that can be seen consistently in terms of outcome.

Less precise and more precise terms can be used in writing objectives to describe behaviors. In striving for precision in program objectives, we may find ourselves in a dilemma. *Flexibility* and *adaptability* are important to health education. The more we are able to adapt programs to meet the

Table 4–2. Precision in Defining Behaviors: More Precise and Less Precise Terms

Less Precise	More Precise
understand	define
be aware of	describe
acknowledge	discuss
feel	answer
know	tabulate
be motivated to	identify
experience	list
be informed of	write
realize	report
be involved in	state

Adapted from: Fodor, J.T., and Dalis, G.T.: Health Instruction: Theory and Application. 3rd Ed. Philadelphia, Lea & Febiger, 1981.

unique needs of individuals, the more likely we are to provide an experience that will bring about change; however, when we emphasize precision in developing objectives, we limit the flexibility and adaptability of the program. We must make an informed choice in program planning as to the desired level of precision and the adaptability of the program to individual needs.[17] For example, an objective such as "at the end of the program participants will be able to list three behavioral correlates of hypertension" may influence some change in behavior, but will not be as effective for the individual as an objective such as "at the end of the program participants will list three personal behaviors that influence hypertension." The former objective specifies program content to include information useful to those with hypertension. The latter objective does not specify content, but rather specifies a flexible approach to each individual in his or her environment.

Another issue that arises with the construction of precise objectives is that of program *generalizability,* or *external validity.* In health education, planners work continually toward developing methods of dealing with target populations effectively that can be applied to more than one setting. We need community health education programs that can be used with different target populations by different health educators and still maintain predictable results. The more precise the program objectives become in terms of one particular target population, the more limited is the generalizability of the programs. When objectives are written with the needs of particular target populations in mind, as we would do to maximize our chances of success, the objectives may not be appropriate for any other population. Thus, the apparent dilemma is how to achieve desirable results within the target population, and yet contribute to the development of health education in other settings. As it turns out, we are most accountable to the clients now served. Out first loyalty in designing community health education programs must be to serve the needs and interests of the current target population.

Measurability. As discussed previously, program objectives should be measurable. Many objectives are criterion-referenced, having a standard of performance that serves as an implicit criterion for assessment of performance. When objectives are constructed with criteria for performance included, the evaluation of the program is helped, but an issue regarding the value of the measurement arises. If an objective is written with a built-in criterion for success, then the assumption is that the program will have served the client properly when the client performs to the standard set by the objectives. To the extent that the standard set by a criterion-referenced objective reflects realistic, useful goals for the client in an everyday living situation, a reasonable standard of measurement is achieved. For example, "by the end of the occupational health program, all employees of local mills who participated will have demonstrated the proper use of all safety equipment located in their work area" is an example of an objective that could be easily measured. If the goal of the program was to have employees know how to use safety equipment, then measurement of skill in demonstration would be appropriate. On the other hand, if the goal of the program was to reduce occupational exposure to hazards, the assumption that demonstrating proper use of all safety equipment indicates changes in everyday behavior would be tenuous indeed.

Objectives should clearly identify characteristics of clients who have been well served by your program. Imagine, for a moment, just what characteristics you would expect to see in a person served by your program if everything went as intended. What would be different about them? Would they know more about their health than a similar person not served by your program? Would they behave in a way more conducive to preserving their health than others? Would their knowledge of their health concerns, attitude(s), and health behaviors all be directed in the same way? To answer these questions, you must have precise, appropriate, measurable objectives that will help you identify (and help others identify) changes in your clients that result from interaction with your program.

Estimating Resources and Constraints

After goals for education are determined, the planning group must identify specific *resources* that exist within the target group and from outside sources that can be used to implement the health education program. Some of the resources needed include money, facilities, voluntary manpower, and political responsiveness. Adequate resources must be available to support the change that is planned.

Constraints, forces that are likely to deter educational goal attainment, must also be determined. These constraints may include many of the items in the resources category, but are seen as potential barriers to program success. Often a constraint is perceived by the planning group as the absence of a resource. For example, it may not be possible to reduce the number of occupational injuries because of a lack of manpower to conduct an employee safety training program. Any force that inhibits the implementation of a health education program can be defined as a constraint.

When resources and constraints have been described, further study of specific issues may be required. It may become necessary to revise the educational goal statements or to rearrange priorities because of an unrealized opportunity or an unanticipated obstacle. It must be remembered that the planning group may find the resources and constraints aspect of program planning to be very fluid. Resources can easily become constraints and, more importantly, constraints can be nullified in many cases. Neither resources nor constraints can be either utilized or affected unless they are first recognized, analyzed, and fully understood.

Identifying Methods and Activities

Up to this point, the health education program plan consists of results of the community and behavioral analyses, program and educational goal statements, resources and constraints, and accompanying objectives for educational goals. The planning group must then determine how the objectives can be carried out. In some cases, the objectives imply the type of method or activity to be used in producing change. In other cases however, the objectives are not sufficiently explicit to specify how change is to be produced within the target group.

Methods are generic descriptions of how change is to be brought about within the target group; for example, mass media and community development are two terms used to describe a host of health education activities. In determining what methods should be used, the planning group should assemble as many different strategies as possible to assure sufficient options.[4, 18] It is essential that the target group be consulted in the selection of the methods to be used. If target group members are part of the planning group, then this consultation process may not be necessary. The planning group must be wary of subtle bias in the selection of methods. Methods are often selected that require little or no retraining for the health professionals, regardless of their usefulness in the particular program. The most important criterion for methods is acceptability within the target population. Some other criteria for selection of methods include literacy of the target population, degree of auditory or visual stimulation in the everyday lives of the target population, customary ways of gaining information, cost of the method, convenience of use, feasibility, and anticipated effectiveness. See Table 4–3 for an expanded list of commonly used methods.

Activities are the specific applications of the methods selected. For example, in selecting a mass media appeal (method), the activity would outline specifically the content and type of approach to be used in the message. Again, consideration of the values, mores, and folkways of the target population is essential to the selection of activities that will produce desired results. Statements describing activities should be sufficiently detailed so that the type and format of the message to be delivered are specified and responsible parties are identified. It is also important that the concept underlying the message be clear. If groups of people are to be educated, the type of leaders and leadership must be specified. Activity statements serve as a schedule for accomplishing the program goals.

Planning Program Evaluation

Objectives that are thoughtfully developed with evaluation in mind are used as the basis for designing evaluation. The extent to which objectives include standards for measurement are expressed with sufficient precision, and are appropriate for the target population determines in a large sense the difficulty that can be anticipated in evaluating the program. In writing the program plan, it is tempting to minimize the need for consideration of evaluation in detail in favor of making certain that methods and activities are selected to provide the best service to the target population. It is always best to consider evaluation in detail during the planning stage, and it may be essential if future funding of a program depends on evaluation. The topic of program evaluation is examined in Chapter 6.

CREATING THE PLANNING DOCUMENT

Producing a written document, a program plan to guide implementation and evaluation, is the final step in the planning process. The program planning document is important because it provides a written record of the program planning process. Such a record can be used by the planning group and other individuals to justify funds needed to implement the program. The written plan is also a guide for program staff during implementation and evaluation. From another perspective, the program plan can draw the target group together, allowing a final confirmation of the identified health needs and goals. The program plan may provide the impetus for the individuals within the target population to organize themselves to resolve their own problems. Program plans generally include seven parts: (1) an introduction, (2) program and educational goal statements, (3) resources and constraints, (4) objectives for each of the educational goal statements, (5) methods and activities, (6) an evaluation plan, and (7) a plan for implementation (Table 4–4).

In some settings, particularly when program planning is conducted by a governmental agency or a voluntary health agency, the format for program plans may differ from that presented here. In addition, other sections, such as a budget section, may be required before a program plan is considered complete.

The introduction to the program plan should orient the reader to the problem to be solved by the program, the target population and why it was selected, relevant descriptors of the problem as experienced within the target population, and a statement of intended outcomes in the target population as a consequence of the program's impact. The remaining sections of the program plan should completely outline the goals of the program, resources and constraints, the objectives for reaching the goals, the methods and activities selected, the evaluation procedures, and plans for implementation.

A health education program plan should be written in a style appropriate for the anticipated readers. For example, a program plan to be read and endorsed by county commissioners would be written in a different style than a program plan used by clinic staff in conducting patient education for hypertensive patients. The most important factor to remember in writing a health education program plan is to write the plan in a style and format so that the plan can be used as a guide in program implementation. A plan that remains untouched on the shelf as the program is underway is of no value at all.

Table 4–3.   A Summary of Characteristics of Commonly Used Health Education Methods

Method	Characteristics
Audiovisual aids (audio: cassette tapes, records; visual: textbooks, charts, posters, diagrams, film-strips, pamphlets; audiovisual: movies, films, slide / tape programs)	Intended for specific audiences, can be used with other methods, impact can be evaluated, requires low to moderate time and involvement from staff and participants, provides modeling, reaches limited number of individuals, used only as a supplement to other methods, must adapt to reading level of audience, practical only with simple health behaviors, promotes only cognitive learning, requires special space, initial and ongoing costs are incurred, low interaction.
Behavior modification (the modification of specific behaviors according to the principles of classical and operant conditioning)	High interaction, has potential for use in clinical settings, based on the concepts of stimulus control and management of rewards and punishments, promotes development of psychomotor skills, can be rigorously evaluated, considered an extreme within health education methods, has not been adequately tested for community use, effectiveness of cognitive behavior modification not extensively documented, requires therapist, requires a highly motivated target population.
Community development (a process-oriented method of community organizing that emphasizes the development of skills, abilities, and understanding in an entire community for the purpose of social improvement)	Works in areas with reconcilable interests and compatible social groups, common use as a health education method, based on self help principles, deals with environmental and economic problems, high interaction, most often used in rural areas, evaluation is difficult, must work with a cohesive group, requires a large amount of time and involvement from staff and participants.
Educational television (use of television for viewing of prepared programs)	Presents self-contained instructional programs, used for an entire class, accepted by educators in school settings, stimulates discussion, saves classroom time, promotes cognitive outcomes, not superior to other methods, effectiveness not adequately tested, requires special space, initial cost incurred, low interaction.
Individual instruction (counseling, patient education)	Personalized, efficient for learner, accommodates individual diagnosis of learning needs, very adaptable for hospital and home use, focuses on cognitive outcomes, accommodates poorly motivated individuals, inefficient for teacher, costly per participant, does not provide for group interaction and support, requires special space, high interaction between health educator and participant.
Inquiry learning (approach in which students formulate and test their own hypotheses)	Focuses on the process of learning, fosters student motivation, develops cognitive skills, promotes affective outcomes, can deal with complex health information, can be used with all age groups, limited effectiveness in the immediate gain of factual information, difficult to evaluate, requires a high amount of time and involvement on the part of the staff and participants.
Lecture-discussion	Easy to use, imparts information, influences opinion, stimulates thought, develops critical thinking, economical, adaptable, practical, can incorporate dialogue be-

Table 4–3. A Summary of Characteristics of Commonly Used Health Education Methods (Continued)

Method	Characteristics
	tween lecturer and participants, involves skills that may be difficult for the lecturer to master, involves participants as passive learners, effectiveness in comparison to other methods is not conclusive, requires special space, labor intensive, provides modeling.
Mass media (television, radio, newspapers, magazines, outdoor advertising, transit advertising, direct mail, telephone)	Can reach large numbers of people, message is self-contained unit, low unit cost, increases knowledge, reinforces previously held attitudes, causes behavioral change if predisposition to such an action already existed, requires little involvement by the target population, does not accommodate differences in audience, difficult to evaluate impact, can present only simple messages, health education messages can often be transmitted as public service announcements.
Organizational development (the implementation of planned change within organizations)	Uses team building, conflict management, data feedback and training; achieves effective working conditions between institutions, agencies and power groups within a community; deals with environmental and economic issues; difficult to evaluate, requires large amounts of time and involvement from staff and participants.
Peer group discussion (Use of small groups for educational purpose)	Suitable for a range of settings, effective in promoting behavioral change, high interaction among all involved, increased motivation, affects attitudes, can deal with complex health information, can be rigorously evaluated, no more effective than lecture in promoting gain of new information, requires high amount of time and involvement from staff and participants, requires special space.
Programmed learning (use of teaching machines, programmed texts, computers)	Presents a complete lesson; teacher often not needed; allows for individual rates of learning; enhances learner motivation; provides immediate feedback to learners; can be used to present straightforward, factual and sensitive information; high start up costs; limited flexibility; can be rigorously evaluated; labor intensive initially, low interaction among participants and staff.
Simulations and games (games, dramatizations, sociodrama, role playing, case studies)	Can deal with complex health information, time and space are compressed, can be used with learners with a wide range of abilities, probably increases motivation, probably has its greatest potential in bringing about change in the affective domain, utilizes experimental learning procedures, related most often to cognitive skills, not currently used widely by health educators, difficult to evaluate, requires high amount of time and involvement from staff and participants, requires special space arrangements, labor intensive, encourages high interaction among all involved.
Skill development (development of specific psychomotor competencies)	Explains need for a procedure and how it is done, demonstrates procedures to entire group, provides opportunities for learner to practice skills, used to improve communication skills through psychomotor development, can be rigorously evaluated, requires large

Table 4-3.   A Summary of Characteristics of Commonly Used Health Education Methods (Continued)

Method	Characteristics
	amounts of time and involvement from staff and participants, requires special space arrangements.
Social action (a mode of community organizing in which a disadvantaged segment of a population organizes to make demands for a redistribution of resources)	Consensus does not have to exist among social classes in the community; deals with environmental and economic problems; not often used by health educators since it represents a departure from their philosophies, skills or mandates; difficult to evaluate; requires high amounts of time and involvement from staff and participants.
Social planning (the process by which experts solve social problems through rational deliberation and change controlled by experts)	Uses rational problem solving techniques, achievement of goals within an institutional context, deals with environmental and economic problems, can be effective with poorly integrated groups, difficult to evaluate, requires high amount of time and involvement from staff and target population.

Adapted from: Green, L.W., Kreuter, M.W., Deeds, S.G. and Partridge, K.B.: Health Education Planning: A Diagnostic Approach. Palo Alto, California. Mayfield, 1980, pp. 86–115.

Table 4–4. Outline for Plans for Health Education or Promotion Programs

I. Introduction
    A. Problem to be addressed by the program
    B. Target population description
    C. Description of the problem(s) of the target population
    D. Intended outcomes of the program
II. Goals
    A. Program goal statement(s)
    B. Educational goal statement(s)
III. Resources and constraints
    A. Available resources
    B. Current contraints on the program
IV. Objectives
V. Methods and activities
VI. Implementation plan
VII. Evaluation plan

EXAMPLES OF PROGRAM PLANS

Five different sketches of program plans are subsequently outlined. The examples illustrate the variety of issues and problems faced by health professionals in everyday practice of planning programs. Different settings are included as are different approaches to solutions of problems. The formats of the plans also vary slightly, reflecting the flexibility of the planning model.

These examples are hypothetical and are intended to illustrate use of the aforementioned planning model. They are by no means complete, but all provide a skeletal framework that can be used as bases for developing the detailed information that would be needed in planning a health education and promotion plan for a specific target population.

Implementation and evaluation are complex topics. They are discussed thoroughly in Chapters 5 and 6, respectively, and for this reason are not included in the program plans that follow.

1. Community-based Education and Promotion for Cancer Prevention
    This program plan addresses a common concern of health professionals in many communities, persuading the public to avail themselves of cancer screening. Medical science has led to the development of useful screening techniques for cancer of the cervix (Pap smear), breast (breast examination and mammography), and colon-rectum (stool guaiac cards and sigmoidoscopy). In using these tests, doctors can detect cancer early in its course, when treatment is most effective. Unfortunately, many people do not undergo screening and suffer the consequences. This plan is for a program to educate the public about cancer screening and to promote wider application of the tests.

    I. Introduction
        A. Problem to be solved: Unacceptable levels of cervical, breast, and colorectal cancers in the target population thought to be associated with low usage of screening tests
        B. Target population: All adult community residents
        C. Intended outcomes: For residents to seek cancer screening tests from the health care system in the community

II. Goals
    A. Program goal: To increase the proportion of community residents who are appropriately screened for cancer
    B. Educational goals:
        1. community residents will learn the value of early detection of cancer
        2. community residents will learn where screening can be obtained and the costs involved
        3. community residents will become motivated to seek cancer screening

III. Objectives
    As assessed by random-digit-dialed telephone surveys, after the program has been implemented community residents will be able to:
        1. describe the relationship between early detection and successful treatment of cancer
        2. recognize the names of the types of available screening tests for cancer
        3. list two local sources where screening tests may be obtained
        4. report their screening status and state when they will need further screening

IV. Resources and constraints
    A. Resources
        1. program staff
        2. local media
            a. television stations
            b. radio stations
            c. newspapers
        3. service clubs that hold regular meetings
    B. Constraints
        1. limited funding making purchase of commercial advertising impossible; Public Service Announcements (PSA) are aired at the discretion of the media
        2. limited staff experience in media relations
        3. local media do not reach all community residents
        4. fear of cancer and mistrust of medical care system at various levels in the community

V. Methods and activities
    A. Methods
        1. communication via mass media
        2. lecture-discussion with audiovisual aids
    B. Activities
        1. develop 30-second PSAs for distribution to local radio and television stations
        2. develop lesson plans to be used in presentations to local clubs and service organizations
        3. develop a schedule for delivery of messages to local clubs and service organizations
        4. develop a network for referral of individuals wanting screening

2. Health Promotion for Prevention of Heart Disease in a Small Community

This health education and promotion program plan identifies heart disease, a significant health problem in many communities, and presents a typical response to the health promotion problem of increasing participation in services that are already available. The plan identifies the target population and subpopulations in need, and is based on the premise that increased participation in services by the members of the target populations will be paralleled by a decrease in early deaths from heart disease.

This program utilizes multiple approaches to promote health. These approaches include increasing services, training community leaders, utilizing interagency resources, and educating members of the target population. The program objectives indicate that changes are anticipated in both knowledge and behavior among the target population.

The program plan could be strengthened by specifying in the program goal and objectives the amount of increase in participation expected as a result of the program. The plan should also include more details related to the needs of the subpopulations and to outreach strategies.

I. Introduction
    A. Problem to be solved: The lack of participation in public health programs designed to prevent early death from heart disease
    B. Target population: The entire population of this small community. Specific subpopulations to receive specific attention include all men over the age of 54 years, and black men in particular

C. Intended outcomes: Increased participation in screening clinics for chronic disease and increased knowledge of the dangers of undetected heart disease

II. Goals

A. Program goal: Community residents, and particularly men age 55 years and over, will increase their participation in screening clinics for heart disease sponsored by the health department

B. Educational goals:
1. community residents will learn of the dangers of undetected high blood pressure
2. community residents with high blood pressure will actively participate in screening clinics
3. community residents will learn about identification of personal risk factors of heart disease

III. Objectives
1. by April 1, community leaders will be trained in teaching of senior citizens about factors associated with heart disease
2. by April 1, community leaders will be trained by public health personnel to take blood pressures
3. by April 15, those in the target population will begin participating in the educational program

IV. Resources and constraints

A. Resources
1. verbal support from the local medical association, the community government, leaders in many of the neighborhoods, and other "well-known" community residents
2. health department conducts clinics each Tuesday from 1:00 to 4:30 p.m., and 8:30 to 11:00 a.m. Thursday
3. cooperation assured from local chapter of the American Heart Association
4. the health educator and nutritionist from the health department will be available to work with the program

B. Constraints
1. poverty is endemic in the community
2. median level of education in the community is below that of the state
3. there is no health education in the schools
4. lack of sufficient medical manpower in the community

V. Methods and activities

A. Methods
1. direct teaching of citizen groups
2. one-to-one teaching
3. demonstration

B. Activities
1. design and implement radio spots announcing the program and its goals
2. meet with public health department leadership and staff to explain their role in the program
3. health educator will design lesson plans to be used by community leaders in teaching senior citizen groups about heart disease
4. arrange for duplication of existing educational materials and development of new materials
5. order additional blood pressure testing equipment if needed
6. meet with local transportation services to arrange for transport of senior citizens to clinic

3. Work-site Health Education

This health education program is directed toward those persons in a rural community who might be exposed to crop sprays and dusts. The target population is clearly defined. The program plan includes knowledge and behavior as factors expected to change as a result of the program.

The program is based primarily on information-giving, with an underlying assumption that the increase in knowledge and ability to apply the information at the end of an educational session will have an impact on the incidence of illness. In the goals and objectives, the program plan specifies the overall amount of change anticipated.

I. Introduction

    A. Problem to be solved: The rising incidence of illness among local farmers and their families resulting from exposure to crop sprays and dusts

    B. Target population: Farm families and farm workers who might be exposed to crop sprays and dusts. Approximately one third of the entire population would be included in the target population; all races, sexes, and socioeconomic strata are represented in the target population

    C. Intended outcomes: First, the target population will use the crop sprays and dusts properly. Second, the target population will understand the risks inherent in failure to take precautions to prevent exposure

II. Goals

    A. Program goal: Reduce the incidence of illness associated with improper use of crop sprays and dusts by 60%

    B. Educational goals:

        1. the target population will learn about the health hazards associated with exposure to crop sprays and dusts

        2. the target population will learn how to prevent exposure to crop sprays and dusts, and proper first aid and treatment for accidental exposure

III. Objectives

    A. For educational goal #1: At the conclusion of the program, 85% of the target population will be able to:

        1. list five specific health hazards associated with exposure to crop sprays and dusts

        2. correctly define safe exposure levels for commonly used crop sprays and dusts

        3. name three common sites for exposure on the body and predict the potential seriousness of exposure associated with each site

        4. illustrate symbiotic effects of smoking, medications, and pre-existing diseases with exposure

        5. list eight signs and symptoms of illness associated with exposure

    B. For educational goal #2: At the conclusion of the program, 85% of the target population will:

        1. demonstrate correct use of protective devices to prevent exposure to crop sprays and dusts

        2. evaluate weather and climate conditions for safety in using crop sprays and dusts

        3. list three steps required in protecting people and livestock from exposure

        4. describe proper spray and dust equipment maintenance and use

        5. list first aid procedures for accidental exposure

        6. list two local sources of medical treatment for exposure to crop sprays and dusts

IV. Resources and constraints

    A. Resources

        1. personnel and equipment of the Agriculture Extension Agency

        2. personnel and equipment of the health department

        3. advice and materials from manufacturers of crop sprays and dusts

    B. Constraints

        1. resistance to education among the target population

        2. time—must complete education before crop sprays and dusts are in use

        3. lack of unanimous agreement among authorities about the relationship between illness and exposure to sprays and dusts

        4. protective devices often viewed as a nuisance by the user

V. Methods and activities

    A. Methods

        1. lecture-discussion for objectives where information is to be given

        2. demonstration for objectives describing skill acquisition

    B. Activities

        1. identify target population and decide when education could be carried out for subgroups

        2. design and implement publicity for the program, use mass media, as well as local suppliers of crop spray and dust products as sources

        3. schedule small groups of the target population, or individual farm units if necessary, for education

        4. with agricultural extension agent, design lesson plan for teaching

5. obtain demonstration equipment
6. design evaluation tools for educational sessions and overall program

4. Health Promotion for a Special Population
    This health education program plan focuses on a preventive health behavior, the use of automobile child-restraint devices. By taking advantage of pregnancy as a "teachable moment," the program increases knowledge related to restraint devices and provides practice in their use. The program goal addresses a behavioral outcome, increased utilization of restraining devices rather than a health status outcome. Although the objectives are measurable, none provides an accurate account of the level of utilization.

I. Introduction
   A. Problem to be solved: Lack of use of protective child-restraint devices in automobiles
   B. Target population: Pregnant women participating in various types of classes designed to prepare them for childbirth sponsored by community agencies, local churches, local obstetricians, and the health department
   C. Intended outcomes: Increased use of automobile child-restraint devices
II. Goals
   A. Program goal: To increase the use of automobile child-restraint devices among those in the community with small children
   B. Educational goal: Members of the target group will learn about the need for and the availability and proper use of automobile child-restraint devices
III. Objectives
   A. At the completion of the program, 90% of the participants will:
      1. describe the extent of the current problem of automobile-related accidental injury and death among children aged 0 through 4 years
      2. explain why special child-restraint devices are needed
      3. list at least three effective techniques for achieving compliance from children in using auto restraint devices
      4. list 6 of the 11 common mistakes made by parents when using devices
      5. describe three factors to be considered in purchasing devices
      6. list at least two local sources for obtaining devices
      7. demonstrate proper use of devices
   B. After the birth of their babies, at least 60% of the program participants:
      1. will give correct responses to a repeat post-test administered verbally by telephone
      2. will indicate verbally by telephone that they are using an automobile restraint device with their babies
IV. Resources and constraints
   A. Resources
      1. available personnel from community groups and professional organizations
      2. supplies available from state organization
   B. Constraints
      1. the cost of safety devices
      2. the limited availability of devices in rural areas and small towns
      3. recruiting volunteers
      4. the amount of time required to train program personnel on the need, use, and availability of devices
V. Methods and activities
   A. Methods
      1. small group presentation and discussion
      2. demonstration of proper use of child-restraint devices
   B. Activities
      1. the health educator will recruit and arrange for training of personnel to give presentations to the childbirth classes
      2. develop lesson plans for presentations using objectives as a guide
      3. the health educator will schedule presentations for childbirth classes and be sure that all parties are aware of and agree to the schedule (plan to have child-restraint device presentation at the end of the classes, i.e., during the last class meeting)
      4. the health educator will secure materials for use in the presentations

5. Staff Education

This health education program focuses on a specific group of staff members as the target population. The program is to bring about changes in attitudes and behaviors among the staff. It is anticipated that these changes will result in an attitudinal change in clients. The program objectives and activities are sufficiently detailed so that measurement of accomplishment is possible.

I. Introduction
  A. Problem to be solved: Lack of teamwork within the staff of a maternal and child health (MCH) program. Other problems related to the lack of teamwork include a high rate of absenteeism, staff impatience with clients, and a high number of complaints made to the supervisor by staff members
  B. Target population: All members of the maternal and child health staff, including the program supervisor, nurse practitioner, health educator, nutritionist, licensed practical nurse, outreach worker, and program secretary. Each staff member expressed a lack of trust for other staff members. Each felt that other staff members were only concerned about their own segment of the program, and cared very little for working toward comprehensive services for the patient. The program supervisor was not able to resolve staff conflict, although individual staff members shared their own feelings with her
  C. Intended outcomes: As a consequence of program inputs, increased staff communication, a lower rate of absenteeism, improved interactions with patients, and increased staff interaction as an interdisciplinary health team should result
II. Goals
  A. Program goal: To increase staff satisfaction regarding individual and team roles so as to have a more positive impact on clients
  B. Educational goals:
    1. program participants will learn role definitions for various team members
    2. program participants will understand the relationship between teamwork and productivity
    3. program participants will understand the impact of poor staff relations on clients and the staff
III. Objectives
  A. By the end of the program all MCH staff members will:
    1. reduce their rates of absenteeism by 50%
    2. report on an attitude survey a 30% increase in their level of satisfaction with their individual roles in the program
    3. report on an attitude survey a 30% increase in their level of satisfaction with interactions within their work team as well as the entire staff
  B. By the end of the program, the program supervisor will have received 60% fewer complaints from staff regarding roles and teamwork
  C. By the end of the year, clients will report on an attitude survey a 40% increase in levels of satisfaction with staff-client interactions
IV. Resources and constraints
  A. Resources
    1. a health educator who is not on the staff will serve as program facilitator
    2. individual staff members each acknowledge the problem and are willing to work toward resolution
    3. available time for inservice training and staff meetings; available facilities
    4. endorsement from agency director
  B. Constraints
    1. heavy clinic schedules
    2. variety of disciplines represented in the staff
V. Methods and activities
  A. Methods
    1. inservice education to include small group interactions
    2. self-study
    3. role playing
    4. use of printed materials and films

B. Activities
1. by January 30, all staff members will participate in a staff meeting in which problems are identified and tentative plans for resolution are suggested
2. by February 28, all staff members will have completed an individual analysis of their own roles as well as their perceptions of roles of other staff members
3. by March 15, all staff members will have discussed their role analysis in a staff meeting; role negotiation will be included as necessary
4. by January 15, a survey identifying patients' level of satisfaction with staff-patient interactions will be designed and implemented; the results of the survey will be shared with all staff members
5. by May 1, a communications workshop will have been designed and presented at four consecutive staff meetings
6. by May 15, the MCH team will have designed a format for their staff meetings that will include at least four of the communication skills learned in the workshops
7. additional training in communications will be given to the maternal and child health program director by May 5

REFERENCES

1. Delbecq, A.L., Van de Ven, A.H., and Gustafson, D.H.: Group Techniques for Program Planning: A Guide to Nominal Group and Delphi Processes. Glenview, Illinois, Scott, Foresman & Co., 1975.
2. Mager, R.F.: Preparing Instructional Objectives. Belmont, California, Fearon, 1962.
3. Making Health Education Work: American Public Health Association, Washington, D.C., 1976.
4. USDHEW, PHS, HRA: Educating the public about health: a planning guide. Washington, D.C., HEW Publ. No. (HRA) 78-14004, October, 1977.
5. USDHEW, PHS, HRA: Bureau of Health Planning and Resource Development, Division of Facilities Development, Committee on Educational Tasks in Chronic Illness: A model for planning patient education. Washington, D.C., HEW Publ. No. (HRA) 78-4028, November, 1975.
6. Weiss, C.H.: Evaluation Research: Methods of Assessing Program Effectiveness. Englewood Cliffs, New Jersey, Prentice-Hall, 1972.
7. Young, K.M.: The Basic Steps of Planning. Charlottesville, Virginia, Community Collaborators, 1978.
8. Silten, R.M., and Levin, L.S.: Self care evaluation. In The Handbook of Health Education. Edited by P.M. Lazes. Germantown, Maryland, Aspen, 1979.
9. Steuart, G.W.: Planning and evaluation in health education. In Behavior Change Through Health Education: Problems of Methodology. Hamburg, Federal Republic of Germany, International Seminar on Health Education, March, 1969.
10. Lieberman, M.A., and Bond, G.R.: Self help groups: problems of measuring outcomes. Small Group Behav. 9(2):221, 1978.
11. Babbie, E.R.: Survey Research Methods. Belmont, California, Wadsworth, 1973.
12. Borg, W.R., and Gall, M.D.: Educational Research: An Introduction. 2nd Ed. New York, David McKay, 1971.
13. Rutter, M.: Community Analysis of Granville County, North Carolina. Unpublished manuscript. Greensboro, The University of North Carolina at Greensboro, 1980.
14. Miller, L.: Principles of Everyday Behavior Analysis. Monterey, California, Brooks-Cole, 1975.

15. Lave, J.R., and Lave, L.B.: Measuring the effectiveness of prevention: I. Milbank Memorial Fund Q., *273*, Spring, 1977.
16. Fodor, J.T., and Dalis, G.T.: Health Instruction: Theory and Application. 3rd Ed. Philadelphia, Lea & Febiger, 1981.
17. Green, L.W.: Evaluation and measurement: some dilemmas for health education. Am. J. Public Health, *67*(2):155, 1977.
18. Green, L.W., Wang, V.L., Deeds, S., Fisher, A., Windsor, R., Bennett, A., and Rogers, C.: Guidelines for health education in maternal and child health. Int. J. Health Ed., *21*(3): Supplement, July–Sept., 1978.

5

Program Implementation

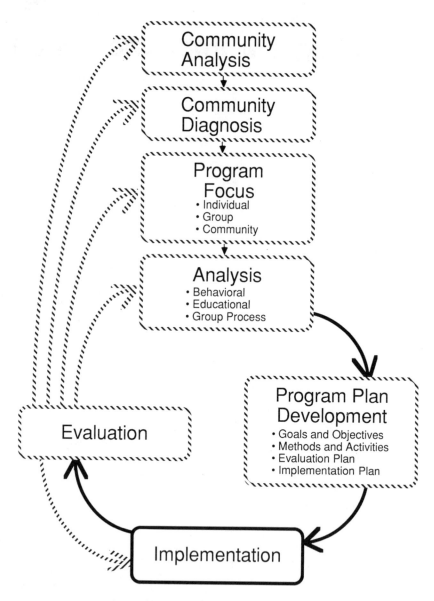

The Health Education / Promotion Planning Model.

5

Program Implementation

As the old saying goes, the proof of the pudding is in the eating. For community health education and health promotion programs, the proof of planning is in implementation—when and how plans are put into effect. The plans include the methods and activities designed to produce behavioral change, and also the procedures to be used for evaluation. A written health education and promotion program plan must include specification of what is necessary to put the program into action. A written plan by itself gives no assurance that a program will be initiated, reach its goals, or be maintained over time. Thus, an essential step in program planning for health education and promotion is development of plans for program implementation. These plans should be included as part of an overall program plan.

The role of a progam planning group may change dramatically during implementation. In some cases, members of the planning group, particularly representatives from the target population, may assume an active role as intermediaries within the target population; others may act as spokespersons for the proposed program. In most cases, however, health professionals must assume leadership roles for program implementation.

In some respects, implementation is the most painful part of the entire cycle, because the time spent in planning may appear to have been wasted due to the large number of changes in the plan that may be required during implementation. When programs are implemented, all assumptions about availability of resources, cooperation of others within an agency or the community or target population, and accessibility of the targets themselves are tested. Not all assumptions necessarily turn out to be correct when the program is actually put into effect. Because of the realities of moment, many programs are changed slightly, and some are changed radically during implementation. Having to make changes in a program during implementation does not necessarily mean that the plan was improperly prepared or the program itself is weak. Change in programs during implementation should be expected. Developing adequate program plans, including plans for implementation, is essential but time consuming. Planners must allow time for this activity.

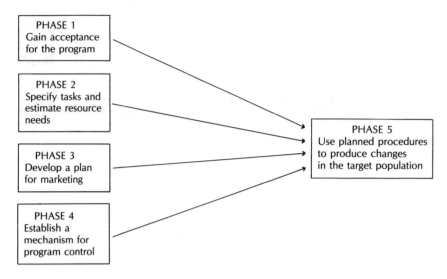

Fig. 5–1. Five phases of program implementation.

PHASES OF IMPLEMENTATION

The five phases in the implementation process (see Fig. 5–1) are gaining acceptance for the program, specifying tasks and acquiring necessary resources, developing a plan for marketing the program, establishing a system for management of the program, and using methods and activities to produce change in the target population.[1] A program plan must document how activities specified in each of these phases will be carried out. A written plan for implementation is particularly valuable in providing guidance to health professionals in the early stages of program initiation.

Although the five phases of program implementation may seem straightforward, health education programs do not rapidly and effortlessly glide through to phase five. Before the target population can be approached about the program as the first phase of implementation, several preparatory tasks must be completed. First, funding for the program must be developed for the short term, and reasonably assured for the long term. Funding is required in part to accomplish the second task, hiring of key program staff. Finally, the program plan must be reviewed by the newly hired staff to acquaint them with the program. Through the course of completing these three tasks, immediate changes in the program that are required for implementation should come to light.

Gaining Acceptance for the Program

Two groups that must accept and support the program before implementation is attempted are the intended target population (consumers of the program) and the sponsors and staff of the program. Because acceptance by these individuals is so important, it is critical that the health professionals planning the health education and promotion program are skilled in working with both the program sponsors and the target population.

Participation of both the target population and the program sponsors in the development of the program plan will help to assure continued acceptance of the program once implementation begins. Additionally, steps of the planning process, such as community analysis, behavioral analysis, and plan development, bring the program sponsors and the target population into continued contact, thereby increasing the likelihood of successful program implementation.

Perhaps most important for implementing programs is an understanding of the relationships between the program sponsors and the target population in terms of power and authority.

Power and Authority

Under most circumstances, an organization does not simply begin offering a health-related service without first having community "license" to do so. License in this sense is recognition from the community or the target population that an organization, person, or whomever has the authority to provide a service. The process through which power and authority are generated is an important consideration for health educators and other health professionals. If they do not have community license to provide health education services, then any hope for success in program implementation is dim.

Power is the "ability or capacity to get others to take steps they would not otherwise take."[1] In other words, power is the clout to get things done. Authority is "the investiture in a position, person, or institution of the means to influence the behavior of others."[1] Stated differently, authority is the means to use power. Power and authority are closely linked. As it turns out, power generates authority, which in turn generates more power, which generates more authority, and so on. This concept is illustrated in Figure 5–2.

Generating Authority. Authority can be generated through extrinsic as well as through intrinsic channels.[1-4]

Extrinsic authority. Authority may be generated extrinsically in two ways—from clients or from the person or agency "doing the job." When authority is generated from clients, that which is gained is a reflection of the power and authority of the client. For example, the Federal government can function as an extrinsic source of authority through law, through funding, and through moral persuasion. Authority is derived when provision of services is mandated through law or when an agency is created. Community Mental Health Centers and Comprehensive Health Planning are two examples. Authority is also generated through funding, which may provide new jobs in communities and new directions for existing agencies. Moral persuasion is often combined with law and funding to produce authority as

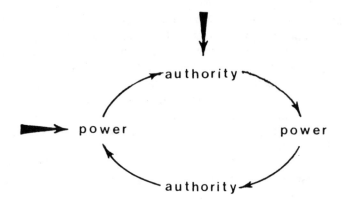

Fig. 5–2.   Power and authority. Power generates authority; authority generates power. Each depends on the other.

in the case of health care efforts directed toward special populations. When government is the primary client of a program, or government creates a program, the authority to initiate processes is implicit.

Authority can also be generated extrinsically through the person doing the job or the organization he or she represents. Acknowledged expertise in an area, employment with an agency that commands respect, and personal reputation all produce authority.[5]

Intrinsic authority. Authority can also be generated intrinsically. That is, authority can be *earned.* When an individual or an agency has a clear record of wisdom and success, authority is created. Positive results from other programs that satisfied most of the target population most of the time generate authority. An ability to understand needs of the target population and flexibility in the face of new information also generate authority. Finally, being of help to those persons already in positions of power and authority, having been of help to politicians in office, and perhaps most importantly, having given the impression of helping the target population serves to generate authority.[1]

In the final analysis, there are two basic considerations to the issues surrounding power and authority relative to program implementation. First, what can having power and authority do *for* a program? Second, what can a lack of power and authority do *to* a program? The answers to these questions are essential in deciding how much authority will be needed in planning for success in implementation of a new health education program for a community.

Program Sponsors

A check for the level of acceptance by the sponsors and staff of the program most often includes both the management level within the organization of the agency that will implement the program and the management of any separate funding agency. In most cases, management gives initial impetus and approval for a program to be planned. Once a plan is developed, management must review and be in continued agreement with the community analysis and the subsequent program plan that spells out activities for the specified target population. Even if the management delegates the responsibility of the health education and promotion program to another health professional, the endorsement of management must continue. Resource requirements, program continuation, and the perceived significance of the health education and promotion program in the broad scheme of services provided by an agency are dependent upon a positive view of the program by the management of the agency.

Target Population

Depending on the level of focus determined for the program (individual, group or community), the program sponsors must be cognizant of issues influencing each of these levels. Four critical attributes of communities or target populations determine strategies for program implementation: local autonomy, coincidence of agency service areas, psychologic identification, and community decision-making.[6]

Local Autonomy. When programs are fully controlled by the target population and those persons sponsoring the programs, implementation is facilitated. To the extent that permission, guidance, or decision-making ability must be sought from sources outside the target population, implementation is impeded.

Coincidence of Agency Service Areas. When delivery of health services, including health education, is highly fractionated with different organizations covering different targets in a non-systematic fashion, program implementation may be impeded. To facilitate implementation, service responsibility should be reasonably apportioned to avoid duplication of effort.

Psychologic Identification. When citizens identify strongly with their community, they are more likely to become involved with health education programs and other community concerns. Program implementation may be impeded if the target population does not have sufficient community identification. When strong identification is not evident, program implementation may be facilitated if the program is able to create a sense of community.

Community Decision-Making and Democracy. In the United States, public health functions through the democratic processes. Measures used by public health officials have been tested repeatedly in both the courts and at the ballotbox.[7, 8] Basic powers given to public health, and others such as police power, have evolved through a long history of litigation.[9] Funding for public health programs is also derived from federal, state, and local representative governmental bodies. Given this heritage, public health programs that come to be implemented would appear to have won approval from the majority. How do we come to this conclusion? Through voting, the will of the majority prevails. Legislators and county officials are elected, and as elected officials they decide whether to fund public health programs, which include health education programs. Therefore, the voters who elected the decision makers do prevail. If the issue in question is subject to local referendum, such as fluoridation of local water supplies, then the "verdict" rendered by the voters seems to bring to bear the full weight of the power of democratic institutions behind the program that has been approved.[7] In many instances, however, particularly in regard to public health programs, those who receive the services of the program do not fully participate in the decision-making process because they do not vote. In many elections, as well as in many decisions made by politicians, those individuals most directly affected by the issue are not represented by the majority of the voters.

If health education programs are designed and implemented with the assumption that the emphasis of public health and the services it provides as mandated by the majority are reflective of the needs of the target population, then there may be trouble with the target population. When members of the target population are not enfranchised, health education programs may appear as being done *to* them, rather than done *for* them. Implementation may be greatly affected as a result. This basic question to be answered is the extent to which the target population participates in local decision-making processes. If the target population does not participate, there may be little interest in the program offerings.

The program plan must be taken back to the target population for approval before the program is initiated. Information about the level of acceptance in the target population is gained through techniques similar to those used in the community analysis. Meetings of selected groups or the planning committees, focus groups, individual surveys, and interviews with key leaders from the target population are a few of the means by which target population acceptance of the proposed program can be checked.

Specifying Program Tasks and Estimating Resource Needs

There are two main ingredients in this phase of program implementation.[12] Program tasks must be *specified* through a detailed review of the program plan. When the program plan has been reviewed and implementation tasks have been specified, the second phase, *resource estimation,* can proceed.

Progam Plan Review

Review of the program plan enables those persons involved with implementation to understand more fully the intentions of the program. This step is essential when there has been a sizable gap of time between the completion of planning and the initiation of the implementation process or when different individuals are involved with planning and implementation.

In reviewing the program plan, three main tasks are to be accomplished: (1) determination of intermediate and final products of the program, (2) preparation of a detailed list of activities included in the program, and (3) listing of the interrelationships among activities.[10] Determining the intermediate and final products of the program helps to clarify the overall goals of the program and the necessary steps in reaching the goals. At this point, the program implementor should make certain that there is no misunderstanding of program goals. Preparation of a detailed list of program activities and the determination of interrelationships among activities greatly facilitate implementation. Of particular interest are those activities that appear to be pivotal, that is, activities that make future activities possible. These activities should be described in great detail to assure their understanding by those implementing the program. The interrelationships among activties can be illustrated in several ways. PERT (Program Evaluation and Review Technique), MBO (Management by Objectives), PPBS (Planning-Programming-Budgeting System), and CPM (Critical Path Method) are methods that may be used to illustrate the relationships among activites, and their sequence in achieving overall program goals.[11–15] Charting the activities has great advantanges in that it allows for anticipation of the usual need for resources.

Determining Resource Requirements

The importance of estimating resource requirements cannot be overstated. Perhaps the most essential ingredient to successful program implementation is having resources available when they are needed. The keys to successful estimation of resource requirements are complete understanding of the program activities, how they are interrelated, and communication with funding sources.

Review of Program Activities. The first step in estimating resource requirements is to review the program activities generated during program plan review. On the basis of this review, minimum staff requirements are generated. Because, personnel costs are usually the largest single part of a program budget, estimating how many persons will be needed and their required qualifications is a vital first task. In addition to estimating minimum staff requirements, customary benefit packages that are routinely offered by the sponsoring organization should also receive consideration.

Consideration of Supply and Equipment Needs. When the issue of staffing has been resolved, or is approaching resolution, the next step in estimating resource requirements is consideration of supply and equipment needs. Referring back to the activities cited in the program plan will generally produce the best estimate of needed supplies and equipment. Be certain to estimate the "lifespan" of such things as audiovisual equipment, and to include maintenance costs and the cost of spare parts for replacement.

Modification of Program Plan. When requirements for personnel, supplies, and equipment have been estimated, the program plan may need modification. If costs of materials have increased since the program plan was completed, the scale of the program may have to be reduced to accommodate scarcer resources. Firm negotiation with funding sources is needed at this point in program implementation, and no steps toward putting the program into action should be undertaken until funding issues are resolved. It may be tempting to put part of the program into action with the hope that additional needed resources will be forthcoming. The pitfall to this strategy is that if a portion of the program is implemented, the needs of organizational administration may be met and further funds may not be made available. It is usually better to hold out for the maximum resource allocation and implement the program as it was designed, rather than approach it piecemeal.

Developing a Marketing Plan

The health professional should consider the target population as consumers of the health education and promotion program. As such, the consumers of the program may need to be convinced of its value to them. The program implementation plan should encompass this concept and include basic marketing considerations; namely the program is a *product* that requires *promotion* to inform the target population that its services can be acquired at a given *place* (or places), at a specific *price*.[17] Consideration of marketing strategies is also advantageous as means for maintaining support of the program sponsors; they too must be "sold" on the program as a worthwhile investment. The health professional or program director should consider the needs of the program sponsors as he or she develops a marketing plan. Internal support is as crucial as the support of the consumers for continued success of the program.

Planning for marketing health education and promotion programs is best carried out by attending to six broad components of marketing plans: (1) objectives that relate to the program's goals in the market; (2) a description of the present and projected status of the program; (3) a list of the possible and desired strategies for marketing the program; (4) a list of staff responsibilities and activities related to marketing; and (6) a list of the specific factors that should be examined periodically as indicators of the extent to which marketing objectives are being achieved.[18]

Establishing A System for Program Management

A system for program management is a set of indicators that is designed to help the program director maintain control over program activities.[10] Two tasks must be accomplished before the system can be designed. Control indicators must be selected or developed, and sources of information for the indicators must be established.[16]

Identifying Indicators

Three basic indicators that can be used to assess program status are time, cost, and performance.[10] There are, of course, many other indicators that may be developed, but most are simple variations of one or a combination of the three basic indicators.

Time is perhaps the easiest control indicator with which to deal. When objectives for programs are stated with time parameters for completion of tasks, series of estimated times for completion of phases of objectives can usually be decided without hesitation. These time "milestones" can then be used to maintain control over program implementation.[15] When milestones are reached early or are not reached at the appointed time, the program director learns of potential troublespots in program implementation.

Another control indicator is cost. Staff time, supplies, and equipment use may be utilized to indicate whether a program is being implemented as planned. Particularly when a program functions on a fixed budget, monitoring costs may be a necessary control indicator.

Performance is perhaps the most difficult control indicator to use effectively. Effective performance of personnel and equipment may be essential to program soundness, but designing performance indicators may be exceptionally difficult. If teaching is a key part of a program, then assessment of performance may be accomplished through informal evaluations or monitoring. Assessment of the performance of program components, otherwise, is difficult. If indicators for performance can be devised and they are judged to be worthwhile, their usefulness to the program director is significant.

Identifying Sources of Information

When control indicators have been established, the next step in devising a control mechanism is to develop a system of data collection that reflects the control indicators' evolution. If any systems for supplying information already exist, they may be used; otherwise, a system for collection of the needed information must be devised. To be effective, any system designed to collect data for program control must be built with the capability of producing valid, reliable information. In addition, the data should be relatively easy to collect, and the act of collection should not have any appreciable effect on workers in the program or the program activities. Sources of information for program control can be identified by using the same conceptual approach used for assessing health behavior. Useful information for program control can be seen as either events or outcomes. It is necessary to select discrete behaviors or chains of behaviors that are necessary for program objectives to be met. It is also possible to select unmistakable results—outcomes of the behaviors—and to use measures of their frequency, duration, sequencing, or absence as indicators of whether program procedures are being implemented as planned.

The following example illustrates how a control mechanism could be designed and used. In Chapter 4, a prepared childbirth program with a component intended to increase the use of child-restraint devices in automobiles was described. How can a control mechanism be established for this program? How can a mechanism be established whereby the progress of the individuals teaching the prepared childbirth classes is monitored? Few systematic behaviors of the teachers could be used to collect control data; however, the resources used in conducting the classes could be considered as an outcome of the completion of a teaching session. A continuing count of expendable resources, such as pamphlets and pencil-and-paper testing instruments could be used as indicators of the number of individuals served by the program. This system would not give any indication of the quality of the presentations, but it would at least provide information on the level of activity. If a means of assessing the quality of the teaching were needed as part of the control mechanism (although this information would probably be considered part of evaluation), spot-checking the pretests and post-tests from a sample of the sessions could determine whether the scores of the participants seemed to be improving. Short of observing the teachers or asking for covert observation of teaching, this would be the extent of the control over the quality of teaching.

Regardless of the system used for program control, the main purpose is to maintain a constant level of service quality and quantity. In addition, control systems allow us to learn of problems as they arise and to devise remedies without delay.

USING PLANNED PROCEDURES TO PRODUCE CHANGES IN THE TARGET POPULATION

The health education and promotion program is intended to bring about specified changes in attitudes, knowledge, or behaviors in the target population. The health professional must keep the change process in mind when planning for program implementation.

Beyer and Trice suggest seven necessary stages for the completion of the change process (Fig. 5–3).[19] Watson, in an analysis of the acceptance of change, categorized factors related to acceptance of change into three broad categories: the initiators of change, the type of change, and conditions conducive to change.[20]

Initiators of Change. When change comes with clear support from the highest authority and the program is coming from within the ranks of the target population and not from outside, change can be facilitated.

Type of Change. When change appears to be reducing the burdens of the target population, agrees with commonly held values, does not threaten security or autonomy, and provides something of interest to the target population, resistance to change is reduced.

Conditions Conducive to Change. When members of the target population have participated in planning for change and the change is adopted

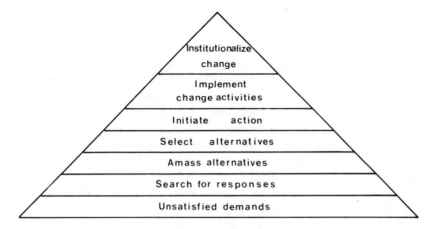

Fig. 5–3. Seven stages in completing change. (Adapted from: Beyer, J.M. and Trice, H.M.: Implementing Change: Alcoholism Policies in Work Organizations. New York, The Free Press, 1978, pp. 22–23.)

by consensus, if opponents have been dealt with empathetically and respectfully, and if supporters of the change understand that misunderstandings of change are likely, the change is likely to occur.

Several concepts of change, put together and presented by Rogers, may be useful when organizing the target population for program implementation (Table 5–1).[21]

A critical step in using the planned procedures to produce changes in the target population is to establish good communication networks among the program director, supervisory personnel, and all other staff members. When all workers are oriented, program activities can begin, and the system for program control can become operational.

Individuals hired to perform a task may be reticent to commit to definite actions until they are relatively sure of themselves. A basic task for the program manager is to design orientation and training for workers so that

Table 5–1. Social Structure, Change, and Social Relationships

1. Social structure acts to regulate the rate of diffusion and adoption of new ideas in social systems.
2. Social structure largely determines acceptance of innovation.
3. Those in power often act to prevent change in social systems while encouraging non-threatening innovations.
4. Top-down change which is initiated by those in power is more likely to succeed than is bottom-up change.
5. Change from the bottom of the social structure involves a greater degree of social conflict than change from the top.
6. Change from the bottom of the social order is more likely to be successful if led by a charismatic leader.
7. The role of a charismatic leader decreases as social movements become institutionalized and more highly structured.

Adapted from: Rogers, E. N.: Social structure and social change. American Behavioral Scientist, *14*:767, 1971.

they may be afforded the opportunity to develop sufficient self-assurance about their jobs before they interact with clients. If this task is not done or is not done well, workers may learn to execute their jobs by using the initial clients as "guinea pigs." This circumstance is unfortunate both for the client and for the program director who wants to see positive results immediately.

What do new workers need to know? They need to know whether they possess the ability to do what is expected of them. They need to know that they can communicate with their supervisory personnel and have questions answered. They need to know the value of the educational products they are delivering and be convinced of their value in a positive sense. Finally, they need to feel they can be successful in their job and that there is a future for them.[10] To satisfy these needs, an orientation and training process should be designed in which the following issues are included:

1. The basis for selection of the target population.
2. The basis for the design of the program including why services of the type used were selected.
3. The objectives of the program.
4. The time schedule for the program.
5. The specific procedures and activities to be used by each worker, including detailed training with "dry runs" to develop needed skills to conduct the program activities as they were planned.

When all workers are oriented and trained, program activities can begin. It is important to remain flexible and ready to adapt, but to maintain awareness of changes as they may affect evaluation and other program activities. When activities are first implemented, they may not proceed smoothly. A new operation requires sufficient time to "work the bugs out," and initial difficulties should be anticipated. When program activities continue to be a source of concern through a reasonable lead-time period, changes should be considered. It may not be easy to distinguish between difficulties that are situational or transitory and will work themselves out with sufficient time, and difficulties that reflect basic problems with the design of the activity or the program. When considerable difficulty with program activities is encountered, and it does not appear that the passage of time will help, the program must be corrected.

It may be necessary to rethink each of the steps in the planning process to identify the sources of the difficulties. Adding new information or making program alternatives to correct the errors made in a step in the planning process should help to remedy problems. Difficulties commonly arise when steps in the planning process were not complete or when significant events have occurred since the planning process was initiated. The steps in the planning process are the basis, or framework, within which to reconsider the specific aspects of the program that have gone awry.

REFERENCES

1. Blum, H.L.: Planning for Health: Development and Application of Social Change Theory. New York, Human Sciences Press, 1974.

2. Boyarsky, B., and Boyarsky, N.: Backroom Politics: How Your Local Politicians Work, Why Your Government Doesn't, and What You Can Do About It. Los Angeles, J.P. Teacher (distributed by Hawthorne Books), 1974.
3. Jones, W.R.: Finding Community: A Guide to Community Research and Action. Palo Alto, California, James E. Freel, 1971.
4. Miller, P.A.: Community Health Action. East Lansing, Michigan State University Press, 1953.
5. Gamson, W.A.: Reputation and resources in community politics. *In* Community Structure and Decision-Making. Edited by T.N. Clark. San Francisco, Chandler, 1968.
6. Warren, R.L.: The Community in America. Chicago, Rand McNally, 1963.
7. Dwore, R.B.: A case study of the 1976 referendum in Utah on fluoridation. Public Health Rep., *93*(1):73, 1978.
8. Hanlon, J.J., and Pickett, G.E.: Public Health Administration and Practice. 7th Ed. St. Louis, Mosby, 1979.
9. Wing, K.R.: The Law and The Public's Health. St. Louis, Mosby, 1976.
10. Bainbridge, J., and Sapirie, S.: Health Project Management: A Manual of Procedures for Formulating and Implementing Health Projects. Geneva, World Health Organization, Offset Publication No. 12, 1974.
11. Evarts, H.F.: Introduction to PERT. Boston, Allyn & Bacon, 1964.
12. Merton, W.: PERT and planning for health programs. Public Health Rep., *81*(5):449, 1966.
13. Moder, J.J., and Phillips, C.R.: Project Management with CPM and PERT. New York, Reinhold, 1964.
14. Roman, D.D.: The PERT system: an appraisal of program evaluation and review technique. *In* Program Evaluation in the Health Fields. Edited by H.C. Schulberg, A. Sheldon, and F. Baker. New York, Behavioral Publications, 1969.
15. Steiner, G.A., and Miner, J.B.: Management and Policy Strategy. New York, Macmillan, 1977.
16. Wolf, R.M.: Evaluation in Education: Foundations of Competency Assessment and Program Review. New York, Praeger, 1979.
17. Lovelock, C.: Concepts and strategies. *In* Health Care Marketing Management. Edited by R.D. Cooper and M. Robinson. Rockville, Maryland, Aspen, 1982.
18. Kotler, P.: Marketing for Nonprofit Organizations. Englewood Cliffs, New Jersey, Prentice-Hall, 1975.
19. Beyer, J.M., and Trice, H.M.: Implementing Change: Alcoholism Policies in Work Organizations. New York, The Free Press, 1978.
20. Watson, G.: Resistance to change. American Behavioral Scientist, *14*:466, 1971.
21. Rogers, E.N.: Social structure and social change. Am. Behav. Sci., *14*: 767, 1971.

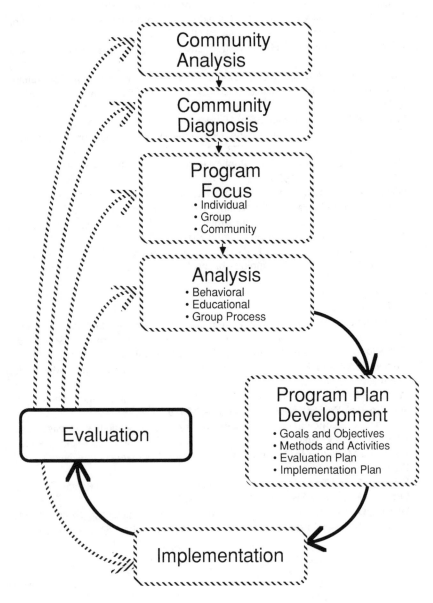

The Health Education / Promotion Planning Model.

6

Program Evaluation

Evaluation is less obvious and is more complex than are the topics discussed in previous chapters. As a result, two separate tasks must now be accomplished. Discussion of planning for evaluation is the ultimate goal, but to understand how to plan, we must appreciate the background and principles that underlie evaluation.

To begin, consider the components of plans for evaluation.

1. Goals and objectives expressed in terms of evaluation
2. Level(s) of evaluation needed
3. Evaluation of criteria for each goal and objective
4. Means of assessment for each evaluation criterion
5. Design of evaluation
6. Data collection plans
7. Data processing and analysis plans
8. Description of the audience for results

This list specifies what is needed for the evaluation phase of the Health Education / Promotion Planning Model. Evaluation is one of the key phases in the model, but it differs from the others in that it also provides feedback for the other phases of the cycle. Stated succinctly, program evaluation reflects not only what happens during implementation but also the basic decisions that were made throughout development.

A working definition for evaluation is the process of inquiry into the performance of a program.[1] This definition includes three concepts that are basic to understanding evaluation.

First, evaluation is inquiry; it is not dictum, controlled by inflexible rules. In fact, as health professionals accumulated experience in planning and conducting evaluations, it became increasingly clear that flexibility is a key element to producing evaluations that address important questions about programs. This is not to say, however, that evaluation has no basis in rules or procedures. Clearly established basic principles should always be used to guide development of plans for evaluation.

Second, evaluation is focused on assessing the performance of a program. Performance may be defined in various ways, depending on the program

Table 6–1. Targets and Types of Evaluation

Performance Indicator	Type of Evaluation
Program development	Formative evaluation
Program accomplishments	Summative evaluation
Processes used by the program	Process evaluation
Impact of the program	Impact evaluation
Outcomes from the program	Outcome evaluation
Experience of program participants	Qualitative evaluation
Count or measurement of experience of program participants	Quantitative (traditional) evaluation

and the motivation for the evaluation. The various definitions of performance in turn define various types of evaluation (Table 6–1).

The third concept is that evaluation is usually based on a standard of comparison.[2, 3] Translating this concept into action is usually one of the most challenging tasks for those planning evaluation, because to be effective, evaluation must focus on a clear indicator of success or failure of the program. The indicator or indicators are developed as an answer to the most basic evaluation questions: What would we expect to observe if the program functioned as intended? The answer might focus on such outcomes as increased knowledge, better access to services, healthier lifestyles, or many other changes, depending on the specific goals and objectives of the program.

SCOPE OF EVALUATION

Purposes

Programs may be evaluated for a variety of reasons.[4] The most commonly cited reasons for program evaluation are to assess accomplishments and to identify limitations. Evaluation can be far from such a sterile, perfunctory task, although it may be used as a method of covertly inducing changes in agencies and / or their programs. In addition, evaluation, which takes time that might otherwise be diverted to other uses, provides additional time for planning. This application of evaluation is particularly useful when little precedent exists for the program and the staff must learn "on the job." Evaluation can also be used to "study" a controversial decision and to divert blame from an individual or agency. This feat is usually accomplished by careful collection, analysis, and interpretation of data that make the decision obvious.

Evaluation is often a necessary part of public relations. Particularly when public funds are used, periodic evaluation may help a program to maintain a good public image and to ensure future funding. Evaluation is also a constant feature of grants. Virtually all grants whether from public or private sources, require some form of structured evaluation.[5]

Finally, program evaluation can be used as a staff development activity. If the staff conducts the evaluation, they may increase their understanding of the program. The result of this process may be renewed willingness to resolve problems.

If a program is being carried out without any clear agreement as to what is to be accomplished, or if there is such strong disagreement with the goals of the program that individuals "do their own thing," evaluation is not worthwhile. When there are no questions to be answered about a program or when decisions about a program have already been made, designing and conducting an evaluation is a waste of effort. Some health education programs are so loosely structured that most activities are improvised and are only guided by the vaguest of objectives. When the program has no clear orientation, evaluation should not be attempted.

Uses

The purposes and uses of evaluation of program accomplishments or weaknesses depend on one's point of view.[6] The major objective for evaluation is to assess what has occurred as a result of the implementation of program plans. A project director may use evaluation as an indicator of the performance of employees or to test the quality of the planning process. From the vantage point of an outside evaluator, evaluation may be used to demonstrate the quality of investment made by private or public sources of funds. To technicians, producers of services, and consumers of services, evaluation may be a more personal matter. Evaluation may mean the loss of a job, a promotion, or a transfer out of a nonproductive program. At this level, evaluation may appear threatening.

Regardless of the point of view taken, several questions are basic to program evaluation:

1. Should this program be continued in its present form?
2. How can practices and procedures be improved?
3. What methods or activities produce the best results?
4. Can this program work in other places?
5. How much money should be spent on this program?
6. Do the results of evaluation support or refute the theory underlying program efforts toward effecting change in the target population?

Because it may present a threat, resistance to evaluation is often encountered. It is rare, however, for resistance to program evaluation to be forthright. Resistance to evaluation is often camouflaged by phrases like "I'd like to be able to explain how this program works, but it's really too complicated" or "we have to improvise a lot because of the varying problems of our clients." When messages such as these are received, the sender may be trying to discourage evaluation. Most do not wish to appear afraid of program evaluation, but wish to avoid being evaluated nevertheless. Part of the program evaluator's "art" is to assuage feelings of trepidation about evaluation.

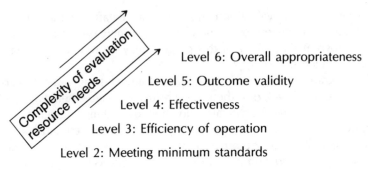

Level 6: Overall appropriateness

Level 5: Outcome validity

Level 4: Effectiveness

Level 3: Efficiency of operation

Level 2: Meeting minimum standards

Level 1: Activity

Fig. 6–1. Levels of evaluation. In general, the complexity and resource requirements increase with the level of evaluation. (Adapted from Blum. H. L.: Planning for Health: Development and Application of Social Change Theory. New York, Human Sciences Press, 1974.)

Levels

Evaluation is normally thought of as measuring the quality of the product compared with a standard: but depending on one's point of view, evaluation can be defined in different ways.[3] Blum cites six levels of evaluation.[7] These levels are arranged in order of difficulty, and also in order of depth of assessment of program accomplishment (Fig. 6–1).

Level 1. The first level encompasses the collection of evidence that demonstrates whether the program is going on. At this level, evaluation is focused on whether personnel are in place to conduct the program and whether the necessary activities involved in accomplishing program objectives are being carried out. This level of evaluation is often used in assessing whether a program is being implemented according to schedule and is followed by more extensive scrutiny of program activities.

Level 2. At this level, meeting standards, evaluations seek to determine whether the program is functioning as designed according to standards. The standards used in assessment on this level of evaluation usually lead to consideration of accessibility of the program to the target population, control over costs, and other criteria that measure the delivery of services.[8]

Level 3. The third level is an assessment of program efficiency.[6] Efficiency is a measure of the cost required per unit of product. In health education programs, efficiency is determined by the provision of planned educational services to a sufficient number of clients utilizing predetermined resources and personnel. The basic questions to be answered at this level of evaluation are whether we are getting what we are paying for. Are personnel functioning at a level at which we can get the benefits we expect? How can efficiency be improved?

Level 4. Program effectiveness is assessed at the fourth level, when the value of the program in affecting change in the target population is determined.[9] If evaluation is to be done at all, and the product of evaluation is to be considered, level 4 evaluation should be selected. Level 4 evaluation asks how well the program produces the desired results and points directly to a corollary question: "How will I know one (a desired outcome) when I see one?"[10] Criteria for evaluation define the designed outcome.

Level 5. The fifth level involves the measurement of outcome validity, i.e., the extent to which the program is successful in dealing with the community health problem for which it was designed. This level of evaluation is truly a reflection of understanding of the problem in the community and asks whether the program produced what was expected.

Level 6. The sixth level addresses the appropriateness of the program in the overall system of health care. This level of evaluation is an assessment of how well the program fits with other programs with similar goals, how well the program fits with the system of health programs in the community, and the extent to which the goals of the program are "good" for society.

These levels of evaluation range from simple to complex in ease of accomplishment, from specific to general in terms of emphasis on program activities, and from nonrigorous to rigorous in assessing the value of program activities. The levels are not intended to be used exclusive of one another; in fact, most community health education programs are evaluated informally on all levels, even if the focus of the formal evaluation is on only one or two levels.

FOCUS OF PROGRAM EVALUATION

Regardless of the purpose or level of evaluation, it should be focused in terms of (1) the type or types of information that will be accepted as evidence of the effects of the program; (2) the role or roles that the results of evaluation may play in the operation of the program; (3) the extent of the need to protect the evaluation from bias; and (4) the type or types of criteria that will be used in the evaluation.

Types of Information

Information that is used to evaluate programs is generally a combination of two types—quantitative and qualitative. Quantitative information is numeric and may include, for example, counts of numbers of program participants, assessment of attitudes, and test scores. Qualitative information is not limited to traditional measurement, and includes formal and informal interviews, photographs, observations of group process, participant observation, life histories, and case histories.

Quantitative evaluation is the traditional approach to inquiry about the performance of a program. It is based on the principles of experimental design and usually has as its emphasis the assessment of performance based on criteria that can be measured with some degree of precision. The goal of quantitative evaluation is to be able to make statements about the probability of the programs producing outcomes in the target population.

Qualitative evaluation is based on some of the same principles as is quantitative, but the emphasis is different. Qualitative evaluation seeks to produce statements describing the processes and experiences that result from participation in the program.

Role of Evaluation

The role of evaluation in the "life" of the program may vary, but two basic roles are implied by the terms formative and summative. Formative evaluation is intended to generate feedback for the development of a program. Summative evaluation is intended to judge the performance of a program that is developed and implemented.[5] Some cross-over may occur between formative and summative evaluation in some instances; the distinction between the two lies in the motivation for the evaluation.

SOURCES OF EVALUATION

Several considerations may come to bear when making the decision between within-agency (or in-house) or outside-agency evaluation. The program administrator's confidence in the validity of the results of program evaluation may be greater when the evaluation is conducted by an outside source. On the other hand, when evaluation is from without, the results are more unpredictable and may threaten the program by exposing weaknesses. Critical issues to consider in deciding whether an evaluation is to be conducted from within or from outside the agency include the following:

1. What are the purposes and uses of the evaluation?
2. Is there anyone within the agency or program who has the skills to evaluate a program according to the designated purposes and uses?
3. Are there sufficient funds within the program to finance evaluation?
4. Are there legal mandates regarding evaluation from the funding source for the program?

Within-Agency Evaluation

When evaluation is conducted within the agency, there is considerable latitude about who in the agency will supervise and conduct the evaluation. For agencies in which a research division exists, evaluation commonly turns out to be one of their responsibilities. When a separate research division does not exist within an agency, evaluation of programs is usually assigned to some part of the administration of the agency. In other cases, the department that actually conducts program activities is charged with its own evaluation. In each of these instances, the obvious question of conflict of interest arises. If the evaluation is conducted from within the agency, care must be taken to remain as objective as possible.

It may be difficult for persons not familiar with an agency to come to grips with its programs. Particularly for programs that are unique, this reason may be used to justify evaluation from within. One of the most common complaints heard from administrators about evaluation is that the evaluation process does not account for the idiosyncrasies of the program, and if the evaluators could only become more familiar with the difficulties the agency has with service delivery, the evaluation would appear much different.

If a program evaluation is to be used to justify changes in which the agency functions, then the evaluation must be defensible. It is very difficult to defend in-house evaluation against the charges of lack of objectivity. For this reason, evaluation designed to make changes in agency function—evaluation designed to eliminate programs or to radically restructure an agency—should almost always be conducted by an outside source.

Outside-Agency Evaluation

Objectivity is perhaps the most commonly voiced reason for using outside evaluation. An evaluation team that is not from within the agency being evaluated will always appear to be more objective about the evaluation than evaluators from the agency itself. Especially when the evaluation is loosely structured and "experts" are identified to conduct the evaluation, the notion of objectivity may be moot. An outside evaluator should have no personal stake in the outcome of the evaluation, and so is usually more concerned with assessing the program according to a set of standards than becoming familiar with the inner workings of the operation.

Several organizations exist that have program evaluation as their sole function. These organizations survive through contracting out their services and conducting evaluations of various programs. Another type of outside evaluation is accomplished through formation of panels of experts who visit programs and conduct evaluations. Most institutions of higher learning, professional societies, and other professional groups use outside evaluation of this type.

CRITERIA FOR EVALUATION

Criteria used in evaluating a program are the standards against which program performance is measured. Standards may be planned into the program as part of objectives; they may be introduced as a result of funding from an outside source; or they may be determined administratively based on agency expectations. Deciding on evaluation criteria is thus a critical part of the evaluation process. In general there are two types of evaluation criteria: criteria specifying effects on *clients* of the agency, and criteria specifying effects on the *agency* itself.

Effect of Program on Client

Perhaps the most common types of evaluation criteria are those dealing with the effects programs have on their clients. In health education, evaluation criteria should be focused on effects on clients.[3] Effects on clients of health education programs include all the different components of behavior change. The evaluation criteria used for health education programs designed to induce behavior change should describe explicit specifications for change in the behaviors of clients. For example, in a health education program designed to increase the use of child-restraint devices in automobiles, the criteria for evaluation might include satisfactory demonstration of proper use of the device, knowledge of common errors occurring with use, and ultimately, regular correct use with the clients' children.

Effect of Program on Agency

Evaluation criteria dealing with effects on agencies are related to institutional changes that have occurred as a result of the implementation of a program. These criteria are usually oriented toward the agency and staff members' relationship with clients. Common indices for this type of evaluative criteria are budgetary changes and "time" changes. An example might be the average waiting time for new patients at a public health family planning clinic after a staff training program. Time changes are changes in the amount of time spent by the agency staff in various functions.

Process, Impact, and / or Outcomes

Regardless of whether evaluative criteria address changes in the client or the agency, all evaluative criteria should deal clearly with process, impact, and / or outcomes. *Process* is the term used to describe the activities of a program that are designed to produce behavioral change(s) in the client. *Impact* is the specific effect on the client resulting from program activities. *Outcomes* are the effects that the impact of the program may have on the client over time.[10] For example, if we consider a program to provide prenatal education, the process would include the activities of the program, teacher-client interaction, reaction of the client to the methods used in the program, and other parts of the program that relate to the "process" of prenatal education. Impact of the program would be the knowledge imparted to the clients by the program, and would include specific facts about prenatal care. The outcomes of the prenatal care program would be the changes in the behavior of the clients after the program was completed, and would be based on the information provided by the program.

Evaluation can be designed to assess process, impact, and / or outcomes. When evaluation is directed toward process, the assumption is that if the process is as designed, then the effect on the client is predictable. For this reason, in addition to the fact that it is often much easier to evaluate process than impact or outcomes, many administrators who ask for program evaluation desire process evaluation.

Impact evaluation is designed to determine whether the methods and activities used by the program result in the desired immediate changes in the client. Impact evaluation is the most important type of evaluation for this stage in the development of health education and promotion and should always be a primary focus for program evaluators.[3]

Outcomes are usually the most difficult to evaluate of the three parts. Evaluation of consequences of health education programs involves follow-up consultation of clients and assessment of their application of the program content. In settings where patients are the program participants and outcomes are clinical entities, evaluation of program outcomes may be a bit easier than in community settings. Ultimately, appraisal of the outcomes of community health education programs—the application of the changed behaviors—is the "acid test" of program efficacy.

How are criteria for evaluation specified? Whether the criteria focus on process, impact, or outcomes, or measure effects on agencies or clients, program objectives specify evaluative criteria.[11] Planning for evaluation as a part of program planning encourages the formulation of sound objectives. If objectives are thoughtfully and carefully developed, evaluation will be facilitated.[6, 10] The clarity of objectives is often tested by their utility in evaluation. Program objectives really specify "how you will know one when you see one."[10] What this phrase means is that objectives really describe the program's products in such a way that an evaluator is able to measure the impact of the program on the person or group. If they are to be useful in evaluation, objectives must specify the specific behaviors or accomplishments to be examined, and how the behavior or accomplishment is to be measured.

MEASUREMENT AND EVALUATION

Evaluation is based on measurement. We cannot evaluate if we do not have the ability to measure. In addition, evaluation is always limited by the precision of measurement. In the most elementary sense, measurement can be defined as assignment of values to objects according to rules. The "objects" can include physical objects, spatial relationships, or abstractions.[1] The rules may be objective or subjective, but they must be consistent. For example, we might measure the effectiveness of a program to promote exercise by the body weights of the participants, the time they spent exercising, or by their perception of well-being. These three types of measurement are clearly different, but each complies with the basic definition of measurement and may provide important information about the program. The type of measurement chosen depends on the criteria selected for evaluation, the need for precision, and the opportunity to collect information. Additionally, the choice is influenced by the characteristics of effective

Table 6–2.   Characteristics of Good Measurement

Sampling	Represents the breadth and depth of what is to be measured. Includes data from all populations to be measured, balances difficulty and complexity of the information.
Communication	Uses units of measurement that summarize the measure effectively and in familiar terms.
Validity	Measures as intended. The object is described through the measurement process.
Reliability	Measures consistently. Measurement that requires little interpretation provides greatest reliability.

measurement: (1) based on a representative sample of that which is to be measured; (2) communicates important information about the program in understandable terms; (3) high validity; and, (4) reliability (Table 6–2).

Characteristics of Good Measurement

Sampling

Program evaluations are based on samples of information. It is not feasible to collect information from every participant or to monitor each and every program activity. Consequently, when evaluation is carried out, it is usually based on a sample of information. The extent to which evaluation is valid is based largely on how well the clients of the program are represented. Clients are not the only focus for sampling, however; program staff, administrators, professionals in other agencies, and relatives of program participants may also be included in the evaluation.

Communication

When the design program for evaluation is begun, the criteria for evaluation draw attention to what will be measured. Depending on the target, "standard" units may be used for measurement. For example, it is widely held that knowledge can be "measured" by the number of items that are answered correctly on a test. In some cases, however, no convenient units are available to be adopted. Regardless, the primary consideration for judging the worth of units that are selected for measurement must include the ability to communicate with others.

Targets of Measurement

An important part of evaluation is the translation of the criteria that can be used to gauge the effectiveness of a program into specific targets that can be measured systematically. The most common targets for measurement include the processes, impact, or outcomes associated with program activities, as well as changes in knowledge, attitude, or behavior of the clients as a result of the program.

Processes, Impact, and Outcomes

Health education and health promotion programs influence target populations through planned activities (process) that may have immediate effects (impact) as well as more long-term effects (outcomes).[3] For example, a program to promote exercise in a community may involve television and radio programs announcing the program's existence and its goals. The impact on an individual seeing or hearing the announcements might be to make them want to learn more about the program. The outcome of their exploration might be a decision to register for exercise classes. For a program designed to teach parents of young children about household safety and accident prevention, the processes might include interaction among groups of parents organized to discuss child safety issues. The impact might be increased recognition of dangerous conditions in the home, and the outcome might be taking action to make changes in the home to prevent accidents and to promote safety. Evaluation can be directed at any one, two, or all of these three components of program effect.

Knowledge, Attitudes, and Behavior

When considering process, impact, or outcome as targets of measurement, we soon come to ask how to focus our attention further so that measurement can be carried out efficiently. The processes, points of impact, and outcomes seldom lend themselves to measurement without clear definition of what is to be measured (see Reference 13). Most health education and promotion programs include specific information, points of view, or recommendations for behavioral change as part of their offerings. Traditionally, we categorize these offerings as knowledge, attitudes, or behaviors. Behavioral change is usually the ultimate goal for health education and health promotion programs. Because such change can be difficult (or impossible) to measure, knowledge and / or attitudes may be used as proxy measures to assess program effects. Although social science teaches that sufficient knowledge and an attitude accepting of change are usually prerequisites for behavioral change, the decision about focusing on attitudes, knowledge, or behavior should not be made casually. In approaching the decision, it may be helpful to develop a flow chart that delineates an idealized path that a client would follow in adopting the changes recommended by the program (Fig. 6–2). As illustrated in Figure 6–2, input of information to increase knowledge and alter attitudes may or may not result in the desired outcomes. We could choose to measure either knowledge, attitudes, or behaviors to evaluate the program, depending on our resources and the opportunity to collect information.

Precision of Measurement

Regardless of the target, measurement processes must be designed to be as precise as possible.[12–14] Precision is expressed in terms of validity and reliability.

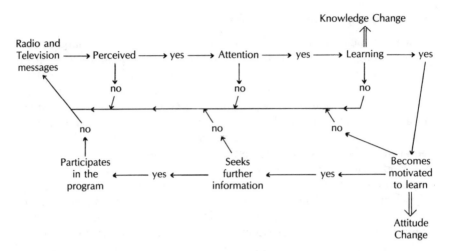

Fig. 6–2. Process of encouraging program participation from mass media messages.

Validity

Validity is the term that is used to express the extent to which a method measures an "object" as intended. A valid knowledge test, for example, measures what is known about a subject. The validity of measurement is based on the type and intended use of measurement. There are three general types of validity; content, criterion-based, and construct. Validity is also oriented in time. The extent to which measurement is valid for present conditions is expressed as concurrent validity. Predictive validity expresses the extent to which measurement predicts future developments as intended.

Content Validity. In instances in which measurement is based on a specific body of information, the validity of the measurement may be assessed by the extent to which the information is represented by measurement. For example, a test to measure what was learned in a work-site health promotion program to reduce the risk of back injury would have good content validity if the information included in the program was sampled in an appropriate manner.

Criterion-based Validity. Measurement can be based on established criteria, such as law or professional guidelines. In this case, the extent to which the measurement process includes the criteria will determine validity.

Construct Validity. Construct validity is the most abstract of the types of validity discussed in this section. A construct is an idea or theme. Self-concept is a good example of a construct. It is common for people to describe other persons in terms of self-concept, but such descriptions are usually based on overall impressions rather than specific behaviors. Measuring a construct like self-concept is, therefore, a hit-or-miss proposition, and validity is more a matter of discussion and persuasion than of fact.

Reliability

The reliability of measurement addresses the issue of consistency. Consistent measurement uses the same processes and generates the same types of information every time it is used. When measurement lacks reliability, we cannot determine whether differences are a result of "true" differences in what was measured or of inconsistent measurement processes.

The concept of reliability is based on the belief that all measurement includes at least some error:

Observed Measurement = True Measurement + Error

Total accuracy exists only in theory. The task of the evaluator, therefore, is to select measurement processes (tests, attitude scales, or behavior inventories) that have acceptable levels of error, and to use them properly.

Discussion of the specific methods of determining the levels of reliability and validity is beyond the scope of this text. Further discussion can be found in references listed at the end of this chapter.

EVALUATION DESIGN

Imagine yourself in this situation. Someone comes up to you in a laundromat and offers you $50 for a dirty shirt that you have in your hand. You accept, naturally. The person pays you the $50 and then tears the shirt in half. After ripping the shirt in half, the person who bought the shirt from you tells you that he is going to show you how powerful his new detergent is by washing one half of the shirt in the detergent you are using, the other half in his detergent. At the end of the wash and dry procedures, he asks you to compare the two halves of the shirt and judge which half is cleaner. Deciding which half of the shirt is cleaner appears to be straightforward, but several issues related to the decision emerge under careful scrutiny of the situation.

First, you must assume that the cleanliness of the shirt halves demonstrates the power of the detergents. If you cannot agree to this assumption, then you cannot proceed at all. Furthermore, you must also assume that the shirt halves were equally dirty before they were washed. If one half of the shirt had grease on it from your car and the other half did not, then comparing the two halves would not evaluate the detergents. Additionally you must assume that there was no difference in the processes used in washing the shirts, i.e., that the two machines used were the same in ability to clean the shirts, the water temperatures were equal, and the cycles were of equal duration and intensity. If you can make all these assumptions and believe that you can really see the difference between clean and not clean with sufficient precision, then you may proceed with confidence.

This situation demonstrates the most basic and important concepts regarding evaluation. The person washing the shirt halves is testing the power of the detergent he is selling. The detergent is an *independent variable.* We can change test detergents at will. The resulting cleanliness of the material washed by the detergent depends on the power of the detergent. Thus, cleanliness is the *dependent variable.* We cannot change the dependent variable except by changing the detergent, the independent variable. That is, what we see or measure in the dependent variable *depends* on the independent variable.

Washing both shirt halves in the same way, except for the different detergents used, provides a standard for comparison. We are using our detergent as a standard for comparison or, in other words, we are using our detergent as a *control.* We can assess any change that is produced by the experimental detergent by comparing the results it produces to the detergent that we ordinarily use.

If we go along with the salesman, and accept that the shirt half washed in his detergent does come out cleaner, then it would appear that his detergent is in fact better than ours. Would this conclusion be applicable to all who washed their clothes in the same way? When we judge an evaluation to be valid and can make all the assumptions reasonably, then we have *internal validity.* Internal validity is the extent to which the results of one evaluation, one episode of washing shirt halves, produces defensible conclusions.

For the salesman to assert that because his detergent worked with your torn shirt it will also work with your pants, underwear, and everything else, the evaluation must have *external validity.* External validity means that the results can be generalized. In addition to the conditions of the washing machines and the water temperatures, there are numerous other factors that must be controlled for the results of this one episode to be generalized. Perhaps the most crucial factor influencing external validity is the extent to which the articles of clothing used in the demonstration of detergent process are representative of all clothing. We did not mention whether the shirt was white, colored, solid, striped, or checked. We also do not know whether this new detergent works as well on blue jeans as on cotton shirts. In other words, we cannot be certain that washing a shirt in any way represents all the clothing with which the detergent might be used. This concept introduces the idea of *sampling.* For our salesman to claim that as a result of his evaluation using your shirt his detergent is more effective than yours for any clothing, he must have picked the shirt from a "universe" of clothing that included all types of clothes in all conditions of "dirtiness." The shirt he bought from you must be a "typical" article of clothing, in typical state of uncleanliness, for his claim of detergent superiority to be valid. The fact that he picked a shirt from you really says that his detergent will clean shirts like the one he bought from you and in similar condition to yours better than your detergent.

The concepts of comparison among elements and groups, manipulation of independent variables, control, and generalizability of results are basic to evaluation design.[13] Whenever we design program evaluation we must take these factors into account.[5, 6, 10]

Design Validity

Several potential pitfalls should be avoided in evaluation design. The goal of evaluation is to collect information that accurately describes the performance of the program. To design an evaluation to reach this goal, the need for internal and external validity should remain clearly in focus. Recall that internal validity is the extent to which the activities of the program were responsible for change that was measured, and that external validity is the extent to which the program can be expected to produce similar effects in different target populations (generalizability). The validity of evaluation is always a matter of debate, so the task of the designer of evaluation is to recognize possible threats to the integrity of the design and to plan to minimize their effect. A useful way to conceptualize evaluation design is to think of the design as a means of eliminating any explanations of the results of evaluation that compete with the "best" explanation—that the results were produced by the program and its activities.

Threats to Internal Validity[5, 14, 15]

History. When events or information outside the program influence the participants, it may be difficult to distinguish between the effect of the program and the effect of the outside information. Evaluation results may be due to the program activities or other outside influences. In practical terms, "historical" influence is difficult to prevent, but it must be recognized and acknowledged as a competing explanation for program effects.

Maturation. People gain experience and knowledge with time. For those cases in which such naturally occurring changes may be confused with program effects, maturation may influence the evaluation.

Testing. When information for evaluation is repeatedly collected from the same individuals, earlier measurements may well influence those that follow.

Instrumentation. If the procedures for measurement change during the course of the program, any differences in the new and old procedures may alter the outcome of the evaluation.

Regression. This threat is most important for evaluations in which the information collected is in the form of scores from knowledge tests, attitude scales, and the like. On any given occasion, any individual is likely to have an extreme performance, good or bad, that deviates considerably from the group mean (average). When retested, the same person would likely perform closer to the group mean, and would generate a score that better reflects his or her true state at the time of testing. Any inference based on the extreme score would be spurious. This phenomenon is also known as "regression to the mean."

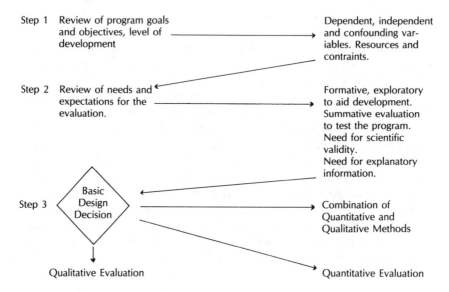

Step 1   Review of program goals
and objectives, level of ——————————→
development

Dependent, independent
and confounding var-
iables. Resources and
contraints.

Step 2   Review of needs and ←
expectations for the ——————————→
evaluation.

Formative, exploratory
to aid development.
Summative evaluation
to test the program.
Need for scientific
validity.
Need for explanatory
information.

Step 3   Basic
Design ←
Decision ——————————→

Combination of
Quantitative and
Qualitative Methods

Qualitative Evaluation   Quantitative Evaluation

Fig. 6–3. Selecting an approach to evaluation design; quantitative, qualitative, or combined.

Selection. Selection poses a threat to internal validity when the difference between groups is due to the particular characteristics of individuals in the groups and not to the program activities.

Attrition. Individuals often drop out of programs and are not available for all evaluation activities. When specific types of people drop out of the program, those individuals who have the most or least to gain from a program or those in one group, the results of evaluation may be uninterpretable.

Threats to External Validity

The generalizability of program effects depends on the ability to transfer program activities successfully into new settings. Naturally, the more a program is tailored to the needs of a particular target population, the less likely it is that transfer will be successful; i.e., the more the methods used are geared to the characteristics of a specific group of clients, the more external validity is jeopardized.

Selecting an Evaluation Design

Selecting an evaluation design involves two basic sets of tasks. First, it is helpful to review the program that is to be evaluated and settle on an overall approach; qualitative, quantitative, or a combination of the two (Figure 6–3). Second, answers to several key questions will help to match the needs of the evaluation with an appropriate design.

1. What is the current level of development of the program? Is it a "new" program that is undergoing change or is it firmly established with all the "bugs" worked out?

2. At what point in time is it or will it be possible to collect evaluation information—before the program begins, during its course, and / or after the program is terminated?
3. What type or types of information can be collected and from whom? Can participants be asked about the program directly?
4. How much time is available to collect information from the typical program participant?
5. Can information be collected from individuals who are not program participants?

QUANTITATIVE EVALUATION

Developing a design for evaluation of a health education and promotion program can be complicated. When the results of evaluation are to be used for decisions about resource allocation or funding, it is wise to seek professional assistance in designing evaluation.

Evaluation of most health education programs can be considered from two basic perspectives.[7] These two points of view about evaluation summarize what is usually sought in evaluating a program—changes that have occurred in an agency or in a client over time, or the more immediate differences in the agency or the client that appear after exposure to the program. The qualitative approach is distinct from the quantitative evaluation, and will be treated in a separate section of this chapter.

Designs to Assess Before-and-After Changes

Evaluation designed to determine changes that have occurred during the course of a program, referred to in this discussion as *before-and-after designs,* are perhaps the most commonly used approaches to program evaluation. These types of designs adhere most closely to classical experimental designs, and in fact are variants of the classical scientific approach. The use of control groups to compare with the experimental or test groups is a feature of almost all designs of the before-and-after type. Two different types of before-and-after designs are subsequently presented but the reader is advised that there are many other designs of this type.

Design #1: Nonequivalent Control Group, Pretest-Post-test.[15] This type of before-and-after design for program evaluation represents perhaps the most common difficulty in evaluating health education and promotion programs. A program evaluator wants to evaluate a program using a before-and-after approach but finds that he or she cannot divide program participants into two groups and *not* deliver program services to one group, i.e., part of the clients of the program cannot be used as a control group. Blocked in this approach, the program evaluator settles on using another group of clients as a control group. Thus, the experimental and control groups are not really equivalent but are comparable. Figure 6–4 illustrates the evaluation

	Pretest Scores	Post-test Scores
Clients in program	A	B
Clients not in program	C	D

Fig. 6–4. Nonequivalent control group; pretest–post-test design.

design. In exercising this approach to evaluation, the following steps are used.

1. Identify the clients who will receive services of the program to be evaluated.
2. Identify a group of clients who will not receive the services of the program to be evaluated, but who are as similar to those in the program as possible.
3. Collect information about the two groups to find out as much as possible about how they differ.
4. Administer the pretest of knowledge, attitudes, and / or behavior to both groups.
5. Provide the program services to the experimental group of clients. The control group does not receive the services of the progam being evaluated.
6. Administer the post-test of knowledge, attitudes, and / or behavior to both groups.

Analysis of data collected from before-and-after designs is a statistical problem that can be approached in various ways; however, discussion of this type of data analysis is beyond the scope of this text. Essentially, if a program produces a difference in clients, the difference should be reflected in the entries in cells A, B, C, and D of Figure 6–4. If the group of clients receiving the services of the program under evaluation changed during the course of the program, then cells A and B should be different while cells C and D should remain nondistinct. Statisticians are trained to examine such data and use the appropriate techniques to determine where differences may exist.

This evaluation design is a typical example of what are commonly referred to as *quasi-experimental research designs.*[16] The term quasi-experimental is used because the clients in the experimental and control groups were not selected or assigned randomly for the evaluation. True experimental designs

	Pretest Scores	Post-test Scores
Clients in program	A	B

Fig. 6–5. Pretest–post-test only design.

	Before Implementation	After Implementation
Clients in the Program		A
Clients NOT in the program		B

Fig. 6–6. Post-test only design for program evaluation.

require random selection and assignment to experimental groups and control groups. By collecting as much information as possible about the two groups (step #3), however, a defense against questions about randomness can be mounted. Particularly if the two groups represent members of the public who participate in a public health program, one can argue that a person "off the street" could elect to be in the experimental program or the control by chance.

An ethical consideration to be applied to this type of design is denying the control group the benefits of the program. This problem can be remedied, although not completely, by providing for the control group to receive the services of the program immediately after the post-test data have been collected.

Design #2: Pretest-Post-test Only. When a control group cannot be used, the before-and-after effect of the program may be assessed by administering a pretest and post-test to the program participants (Fig. 6–5). This approach to evaluation is weak, and should not be used unless no alternative exists.[17] Use of this type of evaluation design will provide data on changes occurring in the clients during the course of the program, but it cannot tell whether these changes were any different from those that may have occurred in the general population.[16] Without a control, there is no standard against which changes can be measured.

Design #3: Post-test Only.[18] In those instances in which pretesting is not feasible or the experience of pretesting will cause problems with the program, post-test only designs (Fig. 6–6) provide a means of collecting information for evaluation. The obvious drawback to this approach is the lack of information about differences between the groups that existed before the program. If the groups are assigned randomly, this design is powerful.

Design to Assess Changes through Time

Changes that occur through time can be assessed most easily through a *time series design.* A time series design seeks to evaluate a program by measuring changes that occur in evaluative criteria over time. There are five basic steps.[15]

1. Design or select an evaluation criterion, or criteria, that can be used repeatedly.
2. Decide or reconfirm exactly to whom the evaluation criteria will be applied. Be very certain that you can always identify the individuals, groups, or population that will be evaluated.
3. Collect at least three measurements of the evaluation criteria before the program is initiated. Be certain that the data are collected at regular intervals and that the same time span, at least approximately, will be available in the future.
4. Be certain the program is implemented. Any changes that may have been made between the time when the evaluation was originally planned and the program was implemented should be noted.
5. Collect measurements of the evaluation criteria at regular intervals after the program has been implemented.

When the time series data have been collected, examination of the data will focus on two main elements: program implementation and changes in the evaluation criteria.

Program Implementation

The first consideration in the examination of time series data, program implementation, seeks to confirm that the program was implemented as planned. It is particularly important to note any modifications to the program that were established after implementation. Such changes are an expected part of health education programming. Any and all modifications to the program, especially those that might have an impact on the evaluation criteria, must be noted.

Changes in Evaluation Criteria

The second consideration in the examination of time series data concerns the evaluation criteria and how data were collected. Any changes in the criteria themselves and any changes in the way data used to effect the criteria were collected must be noted. The importance of this consideration cannot be overstated. The most important component of time series evaluation is consistent measurement of the same criteria. If the standard for measurement changes, and particularly if there are changes unknown to the evaluator, changes brought about by the program may be missed or changes may be false.

Time Series Plot

If the data have been collected consistently by using the same set of criteria or if any changes in criteria or data collection procedures can be rationalized, then the collected data may be examined. Time series data of this type are not easily *analyzed* in the true sense of the word, but they can

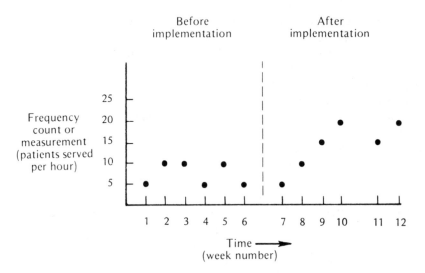

Fig. 6–7. Time series plot of change in clinic patient flow before and after in-service staff education program.

be *examined.*[15] The tool that is used to make decisions with the use of time series data is the *time series plot* (Fig. 6–7). Construction of a time series plot involves the following steps.

1. For each time when a measurement was taken, develop a *summary statistic.* For example, if the measurement was a count of the number of individuals in a clinic waiting room or the number of persons served in a day's time, then the total may be used as a summary statistic. In other cases, it may be more useful to compute an *average* for each measurement interval.
2. Construct a graph with the vertical axis (ordinate) representing the statistic developed in step #1 and the horizontal axis (abscissa) representing time.
3. For each time when data were collected, match the time on the horizontal axis with the amount along the vertical axis. Mark the spot on the graph, and continue for each time period, as shown in Figure 6–7.

The effect of the program on the evaluation criteria can be seen on the graph. If changes in the criteria used for evaluation occurred after the program was implemented, then the data plotted before the program was implemented should be different from the data plotted after the program was begun.

QUALITATIVE EVALUATION

The traditional approach to evaluation is to adapt principles of experimental design, as developed by the "basic sciences," to the needs of program evaluation. These guidelines are intended to control the introduction of factors to the evaluation that confuse the interpretation of results. Properly applied, they function well. The problem with strict adaptation of the principles of experimental design to evaluation of health education and health promotion programs is that the inflexibility that controls for extraneous variation often limits the scope of program activities that can be assessed. The result is that in quantitative evaluations a tendency exists to ignore program effects that cannot be measured with high validity and reliability. What is measured with high validity and reliability may not be important or indicative of the range of program effects. By their nature, health education and promotion programs must have a certain degree of flexibility in order to attend to the needs of clients. The experimental design model does not allow much flexibility. On the other hand, if program effects are not measured with acceptable levels of validity and reliability, and if influences that confound program effects are not systematically controlled, the information that is collected must include the biases of the observer. Greater flexibility is needed.

Qualitative evaluation is based on the need to discover rather than to test the impact of programs.[19, 20] Its goal is to develop an understanding of the processes by which programs reach their intended audiences, the impact that is produced, and the changes that may take place thereafter. Consequently, it has a broader perspective than the quantitative approach.

Qualitative evaluation relies on participants and other persons for information about programs. Because this approach to evaluation is intended to be responsive to individual programs, the methods that are used depend on the situation. Several methods in common use, however, include (1) interviews with those individuals involved with the program, (2) observation of program activities, and (3) participant observation.

Interviews conducted in qualitative evaluation are based on responses to common questions about the program. These questions are usually based on the goals and objectives of the program, but extend beyond to include exploration of "how" and "why" the program activities impacted on the participants. Interviews may be conducted with program participants, staff, or others.

Program activities may also be observed with the goal of discovering aspects of the participants' reactions that are beyond the reach of standard measurement. These observations may be structured to direct attention toward specific behaviors, or loosely structured with little direction.

Participant observation may be used in many forms. Project leaders, group facilitators, or program participants may be the observers. These methods are used to develop a broad understanding of the program from the point of view of the participant.

COMBINED QUANTITATIVE AND QUALITATIVE METHODS

Quantitative and qualitative methods can be used together in evaluation, permitting the collection of information that describes the program in greater depth than would be possible through use of either method alone.[21] Quantitative evaluation emphasizes measurement, ordinarily at the expense of information that is not readily measured. Qualitative evaluation largely ignores traditional measurement in favor of exploration of the meaning of program activities.

If you think of evaluation comprising two primary phases, planning and data collection, the roles of qualitative and quantitative evaluation can fit together in a way that makes sense. In the planning phase, the means for collecting important information about the program must be determined. In typical quantitative evaluations, this determination is constrained by the rules of measurement. Measures should be high in validity and reliability, and should be attuned to the target population. Achievement of these requirements, in addition to the requirement that measurement capture the quantity that is needed to evaluate the program, is extremely difficult. Qualitative evaluation, on the other hand, allows for flexibility in methods for data collection. Therefore, the use of qualitative methods to ensure that the important dimensions of the program are tapped through data collection processes and quantitative methods to ensure proper data collection procedures can produce a superior evaluation.

When qualitative information is acceptable for evaluation, unfortunately, not a common occurrence, quantitative information may be used as a supplement to the qualitative descriptions of the experiences of the program participants. It is more common, however, for the quantitative information to be used to be make primary statements about program efficacy, with qualitative information used to explain why those effects occurred.

As a final note, it is important to acknowledge that the acceptability of quantitative and qualitative information is to a great extent in the eye of the beholder (usually evaluation sponsors). Qualitative information is often seen as "soft" and inconclusive by the technically oriented observer, whereas quantitative information may be inscrutable to the lay reader. Program evaluations may be accountable to either or both types of audience. To ensure effective communication, the design of the evaluation should reflect the needs and interests of the intended audience as well as the goals of the program.

PLANNING FOR EVALUATION

We have established a foundation of information about evaluation. The next task is to answer a series of questions about the program and the evaluation. These decisions dictate the plan for evaluation. The basic questions to be posed and the approach to evaluation (qualitative or quantitative) implied by the answers are listed in Table 6–3. The answers to these questions allow planning to proceed. The planning process can be divided into five steps (Table 6–4).

Table 6–3. Some Basic Issues and Questions about Organizing Program Evaluation

Issue:	Sources of Data
	1. How to identify?
	2. How many or how much required?
	3. How will data be collected? Observation? Questionnaire?
Issue:	Roles for Personnel and Scheduling Tasks
	1. What are the essential tasks?
	2. What qualifications and / or training will be required?
	3. When are tasks to be complete?
	4. How will control over task completion be maintained?
Issue:	Analysis and Report
	1. What analysis will be required?
	2. To whom will a report be given?
	3. Will any extra staff be required to complete analysis or reporting?

Essential Steps

The five essential, basic steps required for program evaluation and their relationship to one another, as shown in Table 6–4, are as follows.

Step 1: Description of the Program and Specific Goals and Objectives. The first step in conducting a program evaluation, whether as an outside evaluator or as a member of the organization sponsoring the program, is to produce a detailed description of the program as it currently exists. The words *as it currently exists* are used intentionally because through time, health education programs tend to evolve. When evaluation is conducted, the program in force may only slightly resemble what was planned originally. Consequently, if evaluation is to determine the quality of the program, understanding of the actual program in force is a basic requirement.

Because evaluation is usually predicated on program objectives, the objectives with which the program operates should be specified before any evaluation activities proceed. At this point, it may become clear that evaluation will not be a worthwhile endeavor because there are no clear goals or objectives for the program or they are so vague that they are not useful.

Step 2: Determination of Criteria to be Used for Evaluation. When objectives are established and the program has been described in sufficient detail to be thoroughly understood, evaluation criteria can be determined. If the program plan was conceived and written with care, then this step in evaluation is made easy. If the objectives for the program were *criterion-*

Table 6–4. Planning for Evaluation: Steps and Products

Steps in Planning Evaluation	Products
1. Clarify goals and objectives	Targets for evaluation
2. Determine evaluation criteria	Standards for comparison
3. Select appropriate design	Approach for evaluation
4. Plan for data collection	Procedures for collection
5. Plan data analysis and reporting	Analysis resource needs

referenced, then evaluation criteria are already established. If the objectives are not written with implicit criteria for evaluation, the criteria must be developed. The key to developing useful evaluation criteria to design them so that no confusion exists about measurement or data collection, and interpretation is clear.

Step 3: Selection of Evaluation Design. After criteria are determined, procedures for conducting the evaluation can be developed. As mentioned previously, many different designs may be applied to the evaluation of health education programs. In developing evaluation procedures, the design of the evaluation must be selected, and all tasks and issues related to conducting the evaluation must be addressed.

The selection of the evaluation design will predict most tasks related to procedures to be used. In addition, many of the questions that arise with the prospect of evaluation will be answered through the design selected. (See Table 6–3 for a summary of basic issues and questions arising from program evaluation).

Step 4: Plan Data Collection. The fourth step in program evaluation is to collect data to assess the extent to which the evaluation criteria have been met. The key to successful completion of this phase of the evaluation is systematic collection of data. Deviations in the way data are collected, or the way in which criteria for evaluation are applied, can destroy the entire evaluation effort, so consistency is important.

Step 5: Planning Analysis and Report. When the data are collected, the procedures specified in step 3 for analysis can be used. The basic question to be answered by the analysis is how the data collected from the program compared with the evaluation criteria. The analysis should point out where the program met criteria for success, and should also identify components that need improvement.

The report from a program evaluation should be organized to explain how the program was evaluated, what questions were to be addressed, and what was the outcome. The intended readers of the report must be taken into consideration when writing the report. Use of technical jargon may be appropriate for some readers, but the report is then unintelligible to other readers. Emphasis on one aspect of a program, personnel performance for example, may be important to some readers whereas another audience may look for behavioral outcomes in clients. It is generally most important to discuss the effects the program had on the target population and the extent to which goals and objectives of the program were reached.

ACCOUNTABILITY AND PROGRAM EVALUATION

... evaluation is like the vermiform appendix: something attached to a system that seems to function fine without it; yet no one seems to know why it has been added. It is noticed only when it causes pain and threatens to foul up the works.

When that happens, it is likely to be cut out! Increased public interest in health promotion and prevention in preference to cure means more critical analysis and more expected accountability for health education.[21]

Accountability conveys the idea of being responsible for one's actions, or "subject to giving an account."[22] The concept of accountability includes four broad areas.[23]

1. All or most education objectives should be stated in behavioral terms.
2. Evaluation should be based on competency or performance.
3. Evaluation is to be limited to that which can be observed and measured.
4. Techniques of behavioral control are to be used to produce changes stipulated by behavioral objectives.

In education, accountability is interpreted to mean that educators and institutions are to be answerable for what their clients learn.[24] In health education and promotion, the concept of accountability extends beyond learning to include behavior. Health education programs that are designed to change health behavior are accountable for the behavioral change planned. Funding agencies, clients, government, and professional constituencies all demand accountability in various forms.

Use of behavioral techniques for behavioral change and insistence on the use of behavioral objectives implies the existence of a "bargain" as the basis for accountability.[25] The bargain comes in the form of predetermined changes to be produced. Accountability has become increasingly important because of "broken bargains."[25] The remedy for these broken bargains in litigation for malpractice or malfeasance is inherent in accountability. "Public accountability demands that social programs be evaluated in order to find out what works and what does not work, and to find the best match between available resources and the programs most likely to have the greatest benefits."[26] Program evaluation can be used as a management tool to enhance effective management and the allocation of limited resources, as well as a means for promoting accountability.

Causality

Central to the relationship between program evaluation and accountability is the concept of causality.[13] Program activities are assumed to be causally related to outcomes. If this thesis is accepted, then through evaluation we can demonstrate the efficiency and effectiveness of program activities, and thus be answerable to clients, funding sources, and ourselves. The more explicit and detailed the objectives, the more complex is the demonstration of accountability. Meeting the terms of explicit objectives demonstrates accountability.[24]

The essence of program accountability is that there is a responsibility by providers to be answerable to their constituency. Program evaluation helps provide the means to be answerable.

Accountability and Community Health Education

The basis for demands for accountability is the idea that planned activities will result in predictable outcomes. Those demanding program accountability assume that there is a causal relationship between program activities and program outcomes.[13] This assumption is the single most troublesome element for demonstrating accountability of community health education and health promotion programs. As stated by Lessinger, discontent about programs comes about because ". . . fundamental theories of learning and of teaching have not yet been established, and we do not really know how to achieve all the objectives we set."[27] In health education, as in most disciplines, we cannot easily demonstrate a causal relationship between teaching and health education outcomes, but an additional factor exists: we cannot guarantee that the services that we provide will always result in desirable health outcomes. Demonstrating accountability for health education and promotion programs, consequently, is a difficult task.[2]

To be accountable in community health education and promotion programs is to be responsive to the needs of clients. Program evaluation provides data that not only *enable* health professionals to be responsive, but also *demonstrate* that responsiveness to the needs of target populations. The essence of accountability, however, is the willingness to modify practices in the face of the results of evaluation. Courage is required therefore to design evaluation that may be critical of one's efforts. The essence of accountability is not to view it as a "vermiform appendix" that has no real function in a community health education and promotion program, but as a means whereby optimal service to the target population may be maintained.

REFERENCES

1. Dignan, M.B.: Measurement and Evaluation of Health Education. Springfield, Illinois, Charles C Thomas, 1986.
2. Green, L.W.: Evaluation and measurement: some dilemmas for health education. Am. J. Public Health, *67*(2):155, 1977.
3. Green, L.W., Kreuter, M.W., Deeds, S.G., and Partridge, K.B.: Health Education Planning: A Diagnostic Approach. Palo Alto, California, Mayfield, 1980.
4. Chelimisky, E.: Differing perspectives of evaluation. *In* Evaluating Federally Sponsored Programs: New Directions for Program Evaluation, 2 (Summer). Edited by C.C. Rentz and R.R. Rentz. San Francisco, Jossey-Bass, 1978.
5. Weiss, C.H.: Evaluation Research: Methods of Assessing Program Effectiveness. Englewood Cliffs, New Jersey, Prentice-Hall, 1972.
6. Rossi, P.H., Freeman, H.E., and Wright, S.: Evaluation: A Systematic Approach. Beverly Hills, Sage, 1979.
7. Blum, H.L.: Planning for Health: Development and Application of Social Change Theory. New York, Human Sciences Press, 1974.
8. USDHEW, PHS, HRA: Educating the public about health: a planning guide. Washington, D.C., DHEW Publication No. (HRA) 78:14004, October 1977.

9. Blalock, H.M., and Blalock, A.B. (eds.): Methodology in Social Research, New York, McGraw-Hill, 1968.
10. Shortell, S.M., and Richardson, W.C.: Health Program Evaluation. St. Louis, Mosby, 1978.
11. Hayes, S.P.: Evaluating Development Projects: A Manual for the Use of Field Workers, Paris, UNESCO, 1966.
12. Cronbach, L.J.: Essentials of Psychological Testing. 3rd Ed., New York, Harper & Row, 1970.
13. Nachmias, D.: Assessing program accountability: research designs. In Accountability in Urban Society: Public Agencies Under Fire. Vol. 15. Edited by S. Greer, R.D. Hedlund, and J.L. Gibson. Urban Affairs Annual Reviews. Beverly Hills, Sage, 1978.
14. Cook, T.D., and Campbell, D.T.: Quasi-Experimentation: Design & Analysis Issues for Field Settings. Boston, Houghton Mifflin, 1979.
15. Fitz-Gibbon, C.T., and Morris, L.L.: How to Design a Program Evaluation. Beverly Hills, Sage, 1978.
16. Campbell, D.T., and Stanley, J.C.: Experimental and Quasi-Experimental Designs for Research. Chicago, Rand McNally, 1963.
17. Dignan, M.B., and Kazanowski, A.: Community Based Patient Education Program. Health Educ., 9(3):10, 1978.
18. Green, L.W., and Lewis, F.M.: Measurement and Evaluation in Health Education and Health Promotion. Palo Alto, California, Mayfield, 1986.
19. Patton, M.Q.: Practical Evaluation. Beverly Hills, Sage, 1982.
20. Patton, M.Q.: Making methods choices. Evaluating and Program Planning, 3:219, 1980.
21. Kreuter, M.W., and Green, L.W.: Evaluation of school health education: identifying purpose, keeping perspective. J. Sch. Health, 48(4):228, 1978.
22. Gove, P.B. (ed.): Webster's Third New International Directory of the English Language Unabridged. Springfield, Massachusetts, Merriam, 1966.
23. Martin, D.T., Overbolt, G.E., and Urban, W.J.: Accountability in American Education: A Critique. Princeton, New Jersey, Princeton Book Co., 1976.
24. Browder, L.H.: An Administrator's Handbook on Educational Accountability. Arlington, Virginia, American Association of School Administrators, 1973.
25. Greer, S., Hedlund, R.D., and Gibson, J.L.: Introduction: The accountability of institutions in urban society. In Accountability in Urban Societies: Public Agencies Under Fire. Vol. 15. Edited by S. Greer, R.D. Hedlund, and J.L. Gibson. Urban Affairs Annual Reviews. Beverly Hills, Sage, 1978.
26. James, T.E., and Hedlund, R.D.: Evaluation and accountability. In Accountability in Urban Societies. Vol. 15. Edited by S. Greer, R.D. Hedlund, and J.L. Gibson. Urban Affairs Annual Reviews. Beverly Hills, Sage, 1978.
27. Lessinger, L.M.: Accountability and humanism: a productive educational complementarity. In Accountability: Systems Planning in Education. Edited by C.D. Sabine. Homewood, Illinois, ETC, 1973.

FURTHER READINGS

Cochrane, A.L.: Effectiveness and Efficiency: Random Reflections on Health Services. London, Nuffield Prov. Hosp. Trust, 1972.

Cook, T.D., and Campbell, D.T.: Quasi-Experimentation: Design & Analysis Issues for Field Settings. Boston, Houghton Mifflin, 1979.

Cook, T.D., and Reichardt, C. (eds.): Qualitative and Quantitative Methods in Evaluation Research. Beverly Hills, Sage, 1979.

Dignan, M.B.: Measurement and Evaluation of Health Education. Springfield, Illinois, Charles C Thomas, 1986.

Effects of restricting federal funds for abortion—Texas. Morbidity and Mortality Weekly Report, *29*(2):253, 1980.

Fetterman, D.M. (ed.): Ethnography in Educational Evaluation. Beverly Hills, California, Sage, 1984.

Green, L.W.: Toward cost-benefit evaluation of health education: some concepts, methods and examples. Health Educ. Q., *2*(Suppl. 1):34, 1974.

Green, L.W., and Figa-Talamanca, I.: Suggested designs for the evaluation of patient education programs. Health Educ. Q., *2*:54, Spring, 1974.

Green, L.W., and Lewis, F.M.: Measurement and Evaluation in Health Education and Health Promotion. Palo Alto, California, Mayfield, 1986.

Hochbaum, G.: Public Participation in Medical Screening Programs. USDHEW, PHS, Publication No. 572, 1958.

Lau, R., Kane, R., Berry, S., Ware, J., and Roy, D.: Channeling health: a review of televised health campaigns. Health Educ. Q., *7*(1):56, Spring, 1980.

Lave, L.B.: Economic evaluation of public health programs. *In* Annual Review of Public Health, Vol. I, 1980. Edited by L. Breslow, J.E. Fielding, and L.B. Lave. Palo Alto, California, Annual Reviews, 1980.

Milio, N.: The Care of Health in Communities: Access for Outcasts. New York, Macmillan, 1975.

Morris, L., Fitz-Gibbon, C.T., and Henerson, M.: Program Evaluation Kit. Beverly Hills, Sage, 1978.

Patton, M.Q.: Creative Evaluation. Beverly Hills, Sage, 1981.

Reisinger, K.S., and Williams, A.F.: Evaluation of programs designed to increase the protection of infants in cars. Pediatrics, *62*(3):280, 1978.

Rosenstock, I.: Why people use health services. Milbank Memorial Fund Q., *44*:94, 1966.

Ryan, W.: Blaming the Victim. New York, Vintage Press, 1971.

Schulberg, H.C., Sheldon, A., and Baker, F. (eds.): Program Evaluation in the Health Fields. New York, Behavioral Publications, 1969.

Schulberg, H.C., and Baker, F. (eds.): Program Evaluation in the Health Fields, Vol. II. New York, Behavioral Publications, 1979.

Shapiro, S.: Measuring the effectiveness of prevention II. Milbank Memorial Fund Q., *55*(2):291, 1977.

Steele, S.M.: Contemporary Approaches to Program Evaluation. Washington, D.C., Capital Publications, 1973.

Suchman, E.A.: Evaluative Research: Principles and Practice in Public Service and Social Action Programs. New York, Russell Sage, 1967.

Tuckman, B.W.: Evaluating Instructional Programs. Boston, Allyn and Bacon, 1979.

Windsor, R.A., Baranowski, T., Clark, N., and Cutter, G.: Evaluation of Health Promotion and Education Programs. Palo Alto, California, Mayfield, 1984.

Wolf, R.M.: Evaluation in Education: Foundations of Competency Assessment and Program Review, New York, Praeger, 1979.

Index

Page numbers set in *italics* indicate illustrations; numbers followed by "t" indicate tables.

Accountability, causality and, 152
  community health education and, 153
  evaluation and, 151–153
Agendas, hidden, 88
Agriculture, in community analysis, 25
Analysis, of target group, 13–14. *See also* Community analysis
Attitudinal factors in educational readiness, 72–73
Authority, extrinsic, 115–116
  generation of, 115–116
  intrinsic, 116
  power and, 115–116, *116*

Behavior. *See also* Health Behavior
  assessment of, models for 61–67
    PRECEDE, 62–64, *63*
      enabling factors, 63
      predisposing factors, 63
      reinforcing factors, 63–64
    SORC, 64–67, *66*
      benefits of, 66
      consequences in, 65–66, *66*
      organism variables, 65
      responses in, 65
      stimulus antecedents in, 64–65
  change in, communication and, 9–10
  maintenance of, 60–61
  target, defining, 58–61
  types of, 58–59
Boundary definitions, community, 23–24
Business and commerce, in community analysis, 25–26

Causality, 152
Change, direction of, 93
  in behavior, communication and, 9–10
  magnitude of, 94
  measurement of, 94–97
  planned procedures to induce, 122–124
  social structure and, 122–124, *123*
  stages in, 122–123, *123*
Climate, in community analysis, 24
Cognitive factors in educational readiness, 71–72
Communication, characteristics of, 7–9
Communication / behavior change (CBC) framework, 9–10
Communication / persuasion matrix, 7–9

Community, functional, definition of, 18
  non-place interactions in, 18–19
  place interactions in, 18
  structural definition of, 18
Community analysis, 12, 17–50
  backdrop in, 24–30
    business and commerce as, 25–26
    climate as, 24
    demographics as, 26–28, 26t, 27t
    geographic identifiers as, 24–25
    information collection for, 24
    social and political structure as, 28–29
  basic parts to, 19
  conceptual definition of, 18–19
  data collection techniques for, 46–49
    community forum approach in, 48
    focus group approach in, 48–49
    key informant approach in, 47–48
    sample survey approach in, 49
  diagnosis in, 13, 41–46, 53–56
    community problem verification in, 54–56
    community state of health, 42
    data collection for verification in, 54–56
    health services pattern in, 42–43
    health status vs. health care in, 43–45
    major issue identification and, 45–46
    steps in, 41
    target population identification in, 41–42
  format for, 19–23, 20t–22t
  health care system and, 34–40
    manpower availability, 35–36, 35t
    service delivery organization in, 36–40, 38t
  health educator in, 17
    role of, 19–20
  health status in, 30–34
    morbidity data and, 32–34, 32t–34t
    vital statistics and, 30–31, 31t
  importance of, 17
  social assistance system in, 40–41
Community decision making and democracy, 117–118
Community forum approach, 48
Control, in evaluation design, 140
Control indicators, 121
  sources of information for, 121–122

Data collection techniques, 46–49
  community forum approach in, 48
  direct observation as, 67–68
  focus group approach in, 48–49
  key information approach in, 47–48
  problem verification and, 54–56
  sample survey approach in, 49
Demographics, 26–28, 27t
  dependency ratio, 27
  educational levels in, 28
  family and household characteristics in,
      27–28
  income and poverty in, 28
  migration as, 26–27
  racial and ethnic groups as, 27, 27t
  sex and age distribution as, 26–27, 27t
Dependent variable, in evaluation design,
    140
Development of program plan, 85–110
  assembling planning group members in,
      87–88
  definitions of components in, 86t
  evaluation in, 98–99
  examples of, 103–109
  identification of methods and activities in,
      97–98, 100t–102t
  specifying objectives in, 92–97
  written, 99–103, 103t

Education, health. *See* Health education
Educational goals, 91–92
  long-term vs. short-term, 91–92
  program goals vs., 91
  resources for, 92
  statements of, 91
  verification of, 92
Educational readiness, assessing, 70–74
  attitudinal factors in, 72–73
  case studies of, 75–80, *76, 77, 78*
  cognitive factors in, 71–72
  components of, 71, *71*
  environmental factors in, 73–74
Environmental factors, in educational
    readiness, 73–74
Evaluation, accountability and, 151–153
  causality, 152
  health education, 153
  components of, 127
  definition of, 127–128
  types, 127–128, 128t
  criteria for, 133–135
  agency effects, 135
  changes in, in time series, 146
  client effects, 134
  process, impact and outcome effects
      on, 135–136
  design(s) for, 139–143
  before-and-after, 143–145
  non-equivalent control group, 143–
      144, *144*

  post-test only, 145, *145*
  pre- and post-test only, *144,* 145
  change-through-time, 145–147
  time series, 146–147, *147*
  selection of, 142–143, *142*
  validity of, 141–142
  external, 142
  internal, 141–142
  focus of, 131–132
  role, 132
  types of information, 131–132
  in development of program plan, 98–99
  measurement in, 135–139
  characteristics of, 136–137, 137t
  communication as a function of, 136
  sampling as a component of, 136, 140
  targets of, 136–139
  process, impact and outcome, 137
  knowledge, attitude and behavior,
      137, *138*
  precision of, 137–138
  reliability of, 139
  validity of, 138
  of outcome, 134–135
  planning for, 149–151
  essential steps in, 150–151, 150t
  qualitative, 147–148
  quantitative, 143–147
  scope of, 128–131
  levels of, 130–131, *130*
  purposes of, 128–129
  uses of, 129
  source of, 132–133

"Felt needs," of target population, 55
Focus group approach, 48–49
Focus of program, 13
"Four Ps" of marketing, 10

Generalizability of program, 96
Geographic identifiers, 24–25
Goals, definition of, 56

Health behavior, collecting data on, 67–70
  direct observation and, 67–68
  role playing and, 70
  self-report and, 68–70, *69*
Health belief model, 6–7, *6*
Health care vs. health status, 43–45
Health education, community, accountability
    and, 153
  definition of, 5
  summary of methods for, 100t–102t
  theoretical foundations for, 6–10
Health educator, community analysis and,
    17
  role in, 19–20
  delegation of responsibility and, 89
Health promotion, definition of, 5
  theoretical foundations for, 6–10
Health services pattern, 42–43

Health status, community, 30–34
  goal of, 92
Hidden agendas, of planning groups, 87

Implementation of program, 113–125
  authority generation in, 115–116, *116*
  community attributes in, 117–118
    agency service areas and, 117
    community decision-making and
        democracy, 117–118
    local autonomy, 117
    psychological identification as, 117
  management system in, 120–122
    indicator identification and, 121
    sources of information in, 121–122
  marketing plan in, 120
  phases of, 114–115, *114*
  planned procedures in, 122–124
  resource requirement determination in,
      119–120
  social structure and change in, 123–124,
      123t
  target population acceptance and, 117–
      118
Implementation phase, 14
Independent variable, in evaluation design,
    139
Industry, in community analysis, 25–26
Infectious diseases, morbidity data and, 32–
    33, 33t
Instructional development, model of, *12*
Intake interview format, *76*
Interactions, non-place, 18
  place, 18–19

Key informant approach, 47–48

Manpower availability, 35, 35t
Marketing, 120
  "four Ps" of, 10
  social framework of, 10
Morbidity data, 32-34, 33t, 34t
  infectious diseases and, 32–33, 33t
  non-infectious and chronic diseases and,
      32, 33t
  occupational illnesses and, 32–34, 34t

"Needs assessment," 17
Non-equivalent control group, pretest–post-
    test, *144,* 145
Non-infectious and chronic diseases,
    morbidity data and, 32, 33t
Non-place interactions, 18

Objectives, 92–97
  definition of, 92
  direction of change specification and, 93
  effective, characteristics of, *95*
  magnitude of change desired and, 94
  measurement of change and, 94–97

appropriateness of, 94–95
  precision in, 95–96, 95t
  time frame determination and, 93
Observation, direct, in data collection, 67–
    68
Occupational health and accidents,
    morbidity data and, 32–34, 34t
Organism variables, 65

Place interactions, 18–19
Planning document, creation of, 99–103,
    103t
Planning group, 86–90
  assembling, 86–87
  hidden agendas of, 87
  orientation of, 88–89
    delegation of responsibility, 89
    role negotiation, 89
  recruitment of, 87–88
  target group members as, 87
  volunteers as, 87–88
PRECEDE model of behavior assessment,
    factors in, 63–64, *63*
Problem verification, basic questions about,
    54–56
  community analysis and, 54–55
  data collection and, 55
Process evaluation, 134–135
Program, 4–5
  focus of, 13
  generalizability of, 96
  goals of, 56–58, 89
  plans for, 5, 85–109. *See also*
      Development of program plan
Program planning, communities and, 11
  definition of 5
  general guidelines for, 1–15
  groups and, 11
  individuals and, 11
  parts of, 103t
  process of, 12–15, *12*
  resources for, 54
  targets of, 10–11

Recruitment, of planning groups, 87–88
Research designs, quasi-experimental, 144
Resource requirements, 118–120
Responses, types of, 65
Responsibility, delegation of, 89
Role negotiation, 89
Role playing, 70

Sample survey approach, 49
Self-report, 68-70
  dietary recall and, 70–79
Service delivery organization, 36–39, *38*
  colleague network in, 36
  hospitals in, 36–37
  local health department in, 37–39, *38*
  medical practice pattern in, 36
  mental health services in, 39

(Continued)
  nursing homes and extended care facilities
     in, 37
  patient referral system in, 36
  rural health or inner city, 40
  voluntary organizations and, 39
Social assistance system, 40–41
Social marketing framework, 10
Social structure, change and, 123–124, *123,*
    123t
SORC model of behavior assessment, 64–
    67, *66*
Stimulus antecedent, 64–65

Target population, 10–11
  analysis of, 13–14
  "felt needs" of, 55
  identification of, 41–42

planned procedures for change in, 122–
    124
planning group membership and, 87–88
program acceptance by, 114–115
Transportation, in community analysis, 26

Vital statistics, 30–34, 31t–34t
  causes of death, 31, 32t
  death rate, 31
  fetal mortality rate, 30
  infant mortality rate, 30–31
  live birth rate, 30
  neonatal death rate, 31
Volunteers, 87–88

Work-related injuries, morbidity data and,
    32–34, 34t
Writing planning document, 99–103, 103t